Heart Path Handbook

An Energy Medicine Guide

for Releasing Patterns of the Ego

from Fear and Anger to Love

for Therapists and Healers

and Health Practitioners

by Robin H. White Turtle Lysne, M.A, M.F.A., Ph.D.

E-copy published by Smashwords, Los Gatos, CA 95033

Hardcopy published by Blue Bone Books,

P.O. Box, 2250, Santa Cruz, CA 95063

ISBN#: 978-0-9778645-5-3 revised ISBN #: 978-1-948675-13-0

Library of Congress #: 2014931941

This book and its contents, as well as Energy Medicine as a practice, are companions to other forms of treatment of disease as well as mental and emotional stresses, and are not meant to replace conventional alopathic treatments. As a pre-preventative strategy for treating illness, Energy Medicine, the use of subtle energy, and Guided Imagery can offer reversal of disease on all levels of a person's life prior to manifestation of an illness in a healthy person.

Heart Path Handbook was written originally to fulfill requirements for my Ph.D. in Energy Medicine from the University of Natural Medicine, Santa Fe, New Mexico, in 2013.

This book is the second in the Heart Path Series. The first edition is called Heart Path, Learning to Love Yourself and Listening to Your Guides.

Contact her through her website:

www.thecenterforthesoul.com

www.bluebonebooks.com

www.robinlysne.com

or Blue Bone Books, P.O. Box 2250, Santa Cruz, CA 95063-2250

Dedication:

To my father, Robert E. Heerens, M.D.

who always supported my work with his love,

intellectual discourse, and humor.

You were fantastic, Pop!

Acknowledgements

The following people supported the development of Heart Path Handbook, without whom, it would not be in your hands. Dr. Mark Smith and Dr. Linda Lancaster formed my dissertation committee at the University of Natural Medicine, Santa Fe, NM. Without their keen eyes and astute suggestions, I could not have produced this book in its present form. Their medical and practical expertise was extremely important for the completion of this book. Also at the University of Natural Medicine, I would like to thank Amanda Coker, who is the anchor and supporter for UNM, and who helped with very practical advice. I would also like to thank Barbara Amita whose suggestions and support as a friend and colleague are invaluable to me and helped me to see the greater whole with fresh eyes. Norma Cordova and Robyn Michele Jones, also helped in creating this book with feedback and inspiration. Originally developed from *Heart Path, Learning to Love Yourself and Listening To Your Guides*, (Blue Bone Books, Santa Cruz, CA., 2007), which in turn developed from my many classes on Spiritual Guidance, and Intuitive Development at The Center for the Soul, Santa Cruz, CA., thank you to my many students. A big thanks to David Whyte, and Eric Schneider, whose Rumi memory banks and insights, filled me with inspiration enough to write my own poems. Finally, and most importantly, I would like to thank my Spiritual Guides, who helped me create Heart Path, especially WuLan, my mentor, comic relief and primary co-creator. My love and appreciation extends to all of you.

Heart Path Handbook

by Robin H. Lysne, M.A., M.F.A., Ph.D.

Table of Contents

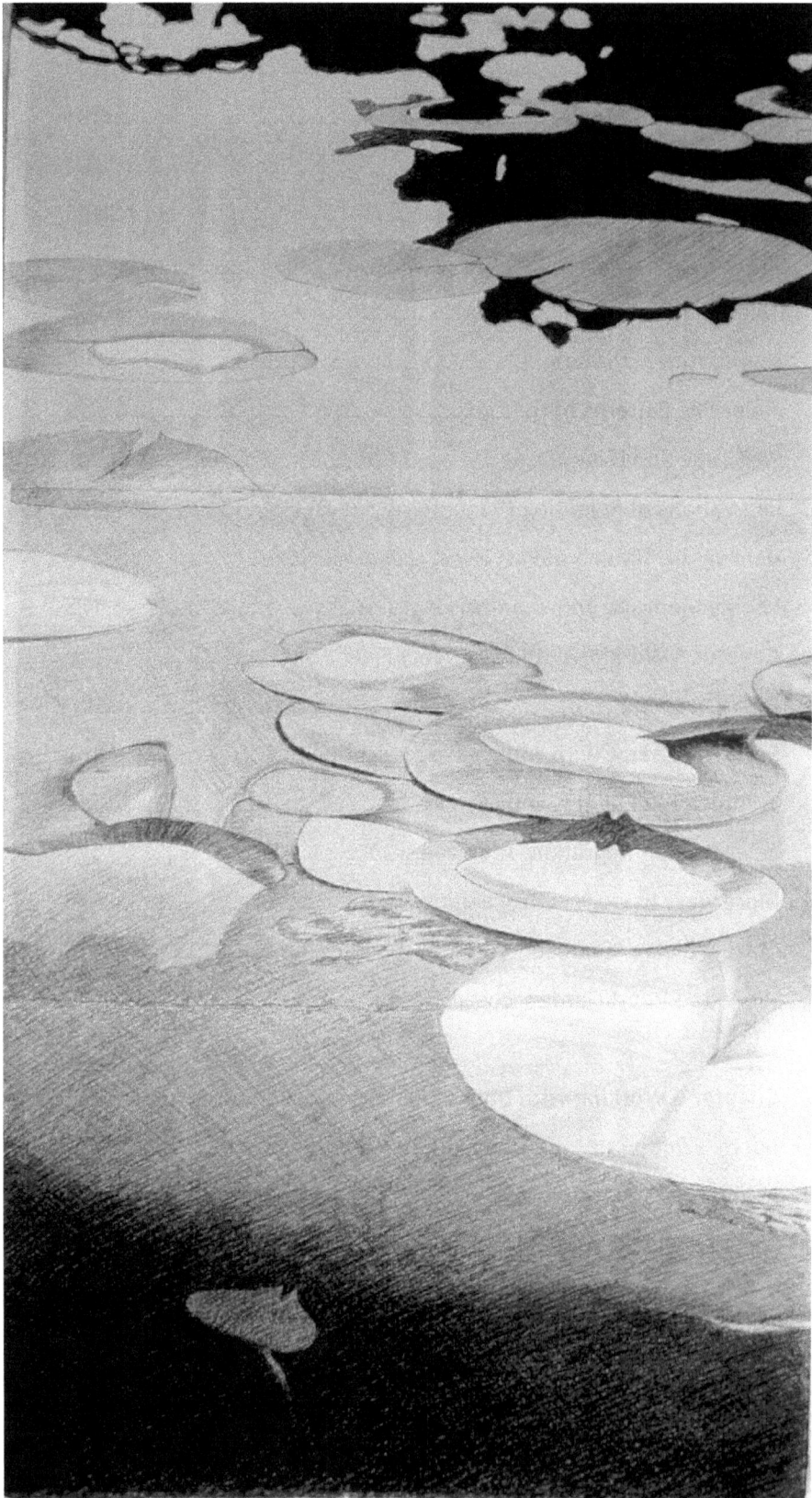

Long Lilies - Charcoal Painting by the Author

Heart Path Handbook

Introduction

<u>Here</u>

Grasshopper, how

easily you rest

across two fern spirals

as though riding

an odd bicycle.

As wheels uncoil

their translucent leaves

the full green plant

rains down the same color

above as below.

You are already in the garden.

Where else

would you want to go?

What is the Heart Path Process?

Welcome to the Heart Path, a guided imagery process that helps people come home to themselves. It supports inner peace, love for the self and harmony as well as safety in the inner work one does inside the self. For some it actually creates an inner landscape they can return to over and over again. It is a path of unconditional love for each one of us if we care to use it, and for one's clients or patients. It begins with the premise that love heals all things, that we are love, and that what is important is for us to be that unconditional love to change the outer world. Heart Path also can help reverse diseases including mental and emotional stress, and conditions that bring pain, discomfort and pathology.

You may be a therapist, healer, teacher and/or visionary, who is interested in transformation. You want to help people move into greater happiness and awareness. You might be interested in your own path of self into Self. In other words, you are interested in ego dissolution or transformation to become unconditional love. You want to transform the ego, and you are here to do that in yourself and perhaps you are here to help others in this very important healing process. You are someone who works on yourself to release the past and be in the present moment with more love and presence. You may feel called to help others from the heart, and in doing so contribute to the support the evolution of all beings. You may not at all be interested in power, but are in the evolution of the self into Self as Love. Knowing that healing yourself is healing the world, you want to make the world a better place.

If any of the above paragraph rings true to you, then this book is meant for you. In fact, anyone who wants to help themselves heal the past, (whether you are a therapist or not) or who wants to follow the path of self-realization, and/or who is interested in being more loving out in the world will benefit by reading this book. These are not mutually exclusive as they are part of the same process towards self-realization. It is a process I have used for over 20 years, with friends, clients, and myself with great success; that is if one defines success as happier people living more fulfilled lives. It is an accelerated path towards self-realization that those of us interested in self-realization are seeking. It is not the only path. As the Persian mystic Jelaluddin Rumi says: *There are a hundred ways to kneel and kiss the ground.* There are a thousand ways to move towards greater awareness.

Heart Path may be the first process that is intended to help people transform the self that also moves one toward full-realization. Even if a client is not interested in Self-Realization, it has become clearer to me working the process of *Heart Path* over the years that clients begin or continue to free themselves from the binds, guilt-trips and limits of the past within themselves and in their relationships regardless of the larger intent of their personal evolution. Clients using the *Heart Path* process have found themselves happier, more free to be ALL of who they are, and more able to express themselves consciously. They may find their faith growing with "the Creator" or with All-That-Is. They may find life more engaging and exciting and they may find that they are much, much happier. They have let go of belief systems that no longer serve them, which is the primary way the ego clings to the past.

They may go through many external changes as a result, however most of the people I work with, are already in the throws of life transitions, and are really ready for internal transformation and change. They are fed up with their lives and are looking for something that can help them complete the process and become more conscious of their negative patterns of relating with others, which no longer work for them.

Heart Path, Learning to Love Yourself and Listening to Your Guides, my first attempt to explain this process, contains the basic meditations and how they relate to our 'energy anatomy', a term coined by Carolyn Myss[1]. I explained how this is connected with the guides, our angels and spirit guides that are with us all the time. I also offered a view of ourselves through the Orixas (elements and combinations of elements, Earth, Air, Fire and Water) and how they can help us become all of who we are. Also at the end of the book were transmissions from the guides that are here to help humanity. As a medium and channel, the first *Heart Path* book, was channeled over six years of classes that I held in Santa Cruz, California from 2001 to 2008. They were held in my home through The Center for the Soul, a place where people came to heal their past and move more fully into the present moment. Star Woman and WuLan were regular teachers who came through my body to speak to the students in the classes.

I wrote the first book with the help of my friend and spiritual mentor WuLan. Like my

---

1   Carolyn Myss, Anatomy of the Spirit, Harmony Books, 1996.

last book, there are places in this book where he is speaking, and are indicated with this symbol (*). He and I shared a past life where I helped him and now he is here to help me. He and I have worked the process with my own issues for several years before we shared it with clients. Since 1995, I have been using it with clients in a variety of settings and have found it quite useful. WuLan brought it through to me from 800 years ago when this form of inquiry was developed in Tibetan Buddhism when he was a Tibetan. I discovered a few years ago that there is an ancient Tibetan tradition of self-inquiry that helps transform the ego that is much like *Heart Path*. This process is called today Bodichitta or enlightenment-mind, also luminous-mind and is a primary way one becomes enlightened in the Buddhist tradition. However, Heart path varies quite a bit from Bodichitta, as WuLan and I incorporated aspects of the human mind that engage the various aspects of the self. These aspects reside in the heart garden while the challenged aspects, or wounded aspects are brought to the outside of the garden to witness, support and heal.

Star Woman is known by Native American tribal people all around the world. She is the darkness behind the stars, the invisible substance of the Universe, that which all substance and creativity comes from. She is amazingly loving and dances when she comes into my body to talk to others. She has brought us the *Three Stars of the Self,* which I will share about later in this book.

Because *Heart Path* is a process that has been given to humanity to help people heal on a soul level coming directly from Divine Guidance, it is very powerful and very simple at first glance. However, this process, though a simple one, becomes more complex as it can be used for many things, depending on one's intention. These different uses are; releasing fear and anger, moving towards forgiveness, present-time healing of relationships, past-life healing, past life-relationship healing, completing with loved ones that are dead, unraveling relationships-especially karmic relationships, or reorganizing them in a more healthy way, rewriting contracts with others, discovering guides and angelic presences. There are also physical pathologies that settle into the body from mental or emotional states, healing physically, mentally, or emotionally are all done with the same basic meditation, however what people experience and how they use the process to heal can look quite different. I also want to pass on the amazing healing gift of Heart Path to those who can use it. These are further reasons to write this book.

Heart Path Handbook differs from the last book because this is a text for those who mainly want to use this process to help themselves and their clients. The Heart Path process is for anyone seeking more understanding about them selves and wanting to heal, however when using it with clients, it is important to understand a few very salient details. While this book further explains the Heart Path process, it also helps a healer or therapist use the process in detail with their clients in a variety of settings. It answers questions that may arise in various client sessions and gives them samples to understand how it might be used for the benefit of all people at varying levels of awareness. It defines and shares some vital information about the ethereal world of Energy Medicine, and helps to clarify terms as well.

The challenge for me in sharing this with you, as the transmitter and intuitive healer working with clients, is that I know every client I work with is different, as every one of your clients are each unique. There is no one-size-fits-all when it comes to helping people heal. Every day I find a new challenge with a client, and every day, I find that these clients are entirely uniquely using the Heart Path process if I have already taught them the process. At the same time, there are structures in the body and in the mind of people that are the same or universal. The Heart Path process accommodates both the unique qualities of each of us while it uses universal imagery and energy to do the transformation.

In meta-physics, (that is the "branch of philosophy that seeks to explain the nature of reality"[2] as in energy medicine) dis-ease comes from the spirit of a person-something their spirit or soul is working on for their life lessons. Then into mental-belief structures of a person or what one 'thinks to be true." Then emotion, one feels to be true-and finally into physical states of being. Heart Path can address all of these levels. By creating a safe space for a client and using Heart Path to witness what is true on a resonant level, identifying life lessons, erroneous beliefs, emotional reactions to things, one can literally dissolve the scaffolding of

---

2   Webster's New World Dictionary of the American Language, Warner Books, NY, NY, 1983.

physical pathology and release the reason for a tumor, or issue in the body that is trying to grab all the attention. It also works in reverse as well and at any point in a person's stressor point. For example if anyone has a tumor already, one can be guided to witness the energy of the tumor and see what it is trying to teach, or say to a person. This does not negate the need for a surgeon, but in some cases it does reverse disease adequately enough and reduce tumor size and in some cases eliminates the tumor all together, avoiding surgery. I will discuss this later in the book.

Because I work from the premise that love, our self-love, heals all things, I know that the love of the self by the client heals their little self into the bigger Self. You may want to know what it is I mean by the little self/ bigger Self.

From a spiritual perspective, the self/Self is part of the same functioning of who a person is, or thinks/feels him/herself to be. What is the personality, the identity, the reactions, the actions, what are the characteristics of a person? All this makes up the self. When the word is capitalized, it refers to the highest potential of a person, not in accomplishments, although that is often expressed as well, but in the most loving, charitable character of a person or the unconditionally loving Self. The Higher Self or Divine Self is an example of Self. When a person transforms the self into Self, one is actually moving a smaller fear-based or anger-based identity with the self into an unconditionally loving identity of Self. The release of ego, that which brings us up or down, occurs. The smaller aspects have been released and the greater loving nature has become identified by the person to be its true nature. There is a dissolving of the old identities and an emergence of compassion. Heart Path gently helps transform the self to Self.

Most people resist this level of healing because they are afraid. They are often afraid of re-experiencing the pain they have already gone through. They think it is narcissistic, or worse they are afraid of being selfish, they are afraid that to love themselves is the last thing they want to do because there is a resistance to loving the adversarial parts of ourselves. In other words, we love to hate those parts we hate. "If only I love everyone else more, then

I will be doing my job," say the females, "If only I can work hard enough and provide for everyone, and be the hero in the family, that will be enough, "say the males. Still they go on hating their very nature. Heart Path can change that so they can love themselves and love others at the same time. There is no conflict loving the self and loving others.

Our work as healers, at least with this process, is to help people (and the masculine and feminine in everyone) meet their resistance gently to assist rebalance through opening to greater self-love. We are the observer and additional witness to their process of witnessing themselves as they heal the past. The compassionate witness—or unconditionally loving presence—heals all things. What I have found is that the client's own self-love does the most good for them. I can offer all the tricks of the trade and my love of them as a client, however, they have to be present with *themselves* in order for the healing to be complete for them. Of course love is our life force energy and it is this fundamental Universal energy that moves through all things. Once we recognize this, we become all we can be—Unconditional Love.

Great teachers and healers have spoken of this level of Self-Realization. Paramhansa Yogananda is one such teacher. He said:

"The ego is the soul attached to the body. Like waves on the ocean, human beings play for a time, caught by the storm of delusion. The ocean, however, is all the time pulling, pulling. Sooner or later, all of them will have to be drawn back, to merge at last into the vast Ocean of Divine Love from which they came. Self-realization is realizing your true Self as the great ocean of spirit, by breaking the delusion that you are this little ego, this little human body and personality."[3]

Healing on the deep soul level that Heart Path addresses, requires the practitioner to be in integrity and focused on their own self-inquiry, dedicated to their own process of Self-Realization. It is not for the faint at heart nor the unimaginative human. This is why medicine and Energy Medicine in particular, is an art more than a science. Healing work requires us to be using our total presence with all of our senses. You cannot do healing work without the senses unless you are simply praying. That works too, however, when one wants to get conscious about patterns so as not to repeat them, Heart Path as a process is very helpful and

---

3   Yogananda, Paramhansa. The Essence of Self-Realization, the Wisdom of Paramhansa Yogananda, Ed. Swami Kriyananda, Crystal clarity Publishers, Nevada City, CA., p. 33

can be an essential tool in dissolving patterns of fear and anger that are no longer useful.

This book is also for practitioners who want to offer deeper work with people. In order to work on a soul level as outlined in this book you must listen to your higher guidance and be in touch with your Higher Self, because we do not, any of us, have all the answers. Connecting with the Higher Self helps you tap into a universal wisdom. You must care about harmony with regards to your integrity. That means you must keep professional boundaries and walk your talk. However you are not alone, and even though each of us may work on ourselves, we have not, any of us, healed all the aspects of ourselves. This is where the guides come in. Our guides can be angelic, religious icons in nature, spiritual Devas, or historic pantheons (Christian, Jewish, Muslim, Buddhist, Hindu, Wiccan, Nordic, Roman, Egyptian, or Greek or you name it). They are here to offer the answers if you listen to them. They will help you stand in your power and integrity for your highest good and they will keep you on track with yourself and with clients. None of us operates in a vacuum. All of us are relational beings. This is why we need to be always listening to the next and the next moment in relationship with others and to ourselves during healing work to offer the best possible treatment. The guides can help us with that too. For me, the Guides are unconditionally loving and deeply caring and right in their approach especially with difficult clients.

Heart Path is initially a path of self-discovery. As another of my teachers (Michael Silverman) has said to me, 'one must have a sense of self before one can dissolve it.' So Heart Path builds the self while it transforms the person from self-loathing to self-loving. It builds to an understanding of the self while the client transforms beliefs and attitudes to more love and harmony. It is also a way of self-transformation that supports self-love. Self-love leads to transformation, which leads to a more authentic nature. If your client is devotional in whatever framework they praise the Divine, whether they praise a form or no form, they are also on the path of Self-Realization at some point in their transformative process.

But I may be getting ahead of myself. *Heart Path Handbook* will begin with some basics and move rather quickly towards a session with a client. I will use examples, changing names, and circumstances to protect identity of those with whom I have worked. In any case, I hope you enjoy it and I hope that you find your work enhanced and encouraged as you move along your path. Finally, it is my hope that you will find new ways to help your clients do the same.

May you discover Heart Path as another tool for your client's welfare. May you help yourself and your clients to greater love that is all around and moving through us. May you receive the highest and wisest wisdom from that Love through me as I write this book.

In flow with All-That-Is,

Robin White Turtle Lysne, M.A., M.F.A., Ph.D.,

Santa Cruz, California

January, 9th, 2014, revised December 13, 2022

Chapter I- Beginning Heart Path

<u>Launch</u>

Jump over those metal fear-teeth.

Dance your way along the ocean surge.

The mountain of your heart

is watching you,

the river of yourself

is flowing on.

Ride the rocket of your longing.

This lake pooling from a rushing stream

beneath this mountain range, only

has an eye for you.

As mentioned before, Heart Path is a guided imagery process that offers the client tools for a lifetime. It works with five basic archetypes that bring together the various parts of our brains and bodies with the archetypes that help us see who we are in the heart chakra, or the center of our being. These archetypes are not symbols of the self—they *are* the self. They are; the inner child, the animal nature, the inner feminine, inner masculine, and all-wise and knowing self or higher self. This makes them different from other archetypes as they are not related to stories. They are our human reality of mother, father, child, animal and higher wisdom self. They help us "see" ourselves not out of an ideal from the past or a fairytale (such as King Queen, Magician, Lover, Warrior) but out of the way it is; Mother Father, Child and Animal Nature and Higher Wisdom Selves. This is why I refer to them most often as aspects of the self, rather than archetypes.

In addition, there are some basic definitions and premises that I work with I would like to share with you before we begin. This is to let you know from the beginning how I work, with what intentions and forethought, so you know my orientation in offering healing work. This may or may not agree with what you have been taught in other schools of healing or therapy. However, I have found them sound when working with others in energetic healing and especially with the Heart Path process. Many schools of healing, psychology and massage would agree. In any case, my guides have been my teachers, along with many here on the ground in bodies and all of them are those that I trust impeccably.

Let's begin by defining healing. This is a word used often by practitioners that can mean a variety of things. In the Oxford English Dictionary the word originates from Old English with Germanic roots from the word "heilen 'to make whole" or "to whole." The contemporary definition "to make sound or whole again" has not changed much from the original Germanic root. So when we are working with someone the assumption is that we are helping to make that person whole again.

From an Energy Medicine standpoint the person is already whole, all the parts are there. In Energy Medicine, a practitioner works with the entire energy of the person, body, mind, emotions and spirit. People offering clients Reiki, or energy work often balance the life force or etheric energy of the person. However, in Energy Medicine, you use your intention and the intention of the client to rebalance and reverse dis-ease and disharmony. Rebalancing the person's field is one thing, intending action with the etheric substance is another. (I will go into more detail in future pages.) The client is in need of bringing what is unconscious to consciousness. When the client consciously brings old patterns and strategies to the surface, they begin to resonate at a higher frequency and become a more *coherent*[4] whole. Coherence allows for a person to resonate at a higher frequency so they get more done, are able to be with the self, feel more at peace, and have more capacity to carry out their life purpose.

Medicine by dictionary definition is; 1. the science or practice of diagnosis, treatment

---

4   Doc Childre, Ph.D., The HeartMath Solution, The Heart Math Publishers, Boulder Creek CA. Doc Childre uses 'coherence' as a way to describe a unified field, and teaches through Heart Math Institute. This is similar to yet different than Heart Path.

and prevention of disease.[5] Because most people come to me with diagnosis already in hand, or a problem they have defined, I try not to diagnose. I never would say to a person, you have cancer or heart disease. I might say; 'let's see if we can reverse this pattern I see in your field.' This way they do not get scared and there is more chance for them to actually heal. If at the end of the session, the energy of the person has not changed, (which has never happened) I would say to them something like, 'and I want to recommend that you check with your physician about this as soon as possible.' If I am pretty positive there is some form of pathology I will ask them to promise me to check with their doctor.

I do practice treatment and prevention of disease. I would say Energy Medicine is the most preventative treatment you could come to experience, as it treats dis-ease when it is in an early stage before it has manifested in the body. Sometimes people come in with physical symptoms such as headaches, nausea, or feeling off. Usually they have gone to their M.D. and the doctor has found nothing or they have already run through a few prescriptions. However, like allopathic medicine, the earlier you treat something the better chance of reversal of disease. In my practice, I try to support the whole person into a resonant whole by engaging their responsibility in the process of wholeness. Also I am engaging them at every level as a whole person, body, mind, emotions and spirit. Often I have people that come to me feeling off, or that something in their system is not right. As we examine the issues in their lives and their process of feeling off, as we look with the heart at the dis-ease, we often eliminate or reverse the illness at its source. This supports the client's resonance into wholeness.

The first realization that I make is that as a "healer" or one who reveals the whole, or supports the resonance towards wholeness, we are not the only ones vibrating towards healing. The client does too. They give their willingness to be brought into coherence and their trust. They bring their story and their beliefs. We facilitate healing by setting a safe space, making suggestions, listening and helping the client sort and address their issues, offering them our awareness and our light and techniques for change. But we do not "do"

5   Oxford American Dictionary, Oxford University Press, England, 2005, pg. 1054

anything that *interferes* with their process unless it is absolutely necessary. We can offer our perceptions and our skills. Our job more times than not is to "be" with them in their process and point things out and help that process along as is needed following the thread of *their* understanding. This is important, because the reality is that the client often knows what they need *if we listen to what they are telling us*, they may not know *how* to do the healing, or what they need exactly, but they know there is something out of balance. How much transformation they can take and what they are able to integrate in any given session is where we come in working alongside them. We can set a harmonious and resonant space for them to come into wholeness. We can help with the *how* and help them identify what needs addressing specifically. Rarely, do I have someone come in who does not tell me in the first few minutes why they are coming in for a session if I am listening. Often they have a very clear agenda if that is only "I had a feeling I needed to come in and see you" or they feel "off". That, in itself, is a pretty clear message.

The process of Heart Path requires trusting the client's higher wisdom and allowing what arises to arise. There is no visual forcing of the images, or 'making it happen.' Heart Path works best if the images just come to the person. Sometimes they don't come readily, so we make a space for those aspects and come back to them. Sometimes they need to recognize more conscious aspects of themselves before they are able to make a safe place for other aspects to arrive or develop. Many times clients subconsciously break off or hide aspects that are 'in danger' when the safety of the heart is not a primary intention with other aspects. For example, a common issue I see often is where the contraction of the lower chakras-- created by a threat or lack of safety by an outside environment or by the client's internal abandonment of presences with the self--creates danger in the body. The spirit of the person ejects up and out of the body. Sometimes the child or the feminine aspects will not appear when the male aspect is too dominant or bossy. They just hide in the aura someplace outside the heart. Sometimes the male aspect is absent if the feminine aspect is too dominant. Healing is achieved when there can be more dynamic balance for the client.

In one recent case, a forty-three year old white female came in with this very condition. In the outer world, every aspect of her life was changing—her job, selling her home (actually two homes) her relationships of those living with her, a divorce—everything that would relate to grounding was shifting. Out of fear she had segmented various chakra levels into emotional reactions at different ages. The two year old lived in the second chakra, the teenager lived in the third, the 18-20 year old was in the heart, the 22 year old in the throat, and the only thing functioning (on overdrive) was the 6th chakra, where her 30 year old was operating in overwhelm, where the sense perception was fearfully looking for the next attach. In one session lasting an hour and a half, which began by her asking me to place my hands on her head to cover her 6th chakra, we brought all the aspects of herself to the Heart Garden one by one, and helped her release belief systems that where holding her back with fear. Over the hour, we released these beliefs; "I have to do it all myself" (2year-old) "I'm not good enough" (12-14 year old) "I can't" (the 18-20 year old), "this is too much" (22 year old) and "I'm overwhelmed" (30 year old). Each of them was integrated into the next, and finally into the inner adult aspects (age 43) and some integrated into the higher self as appropriate. By having the younger age step into the next age into current time we dissolved the aspects towards the higher self. The adult aspects stayed intact and were empowered to function as the adult at her current age. We also helped them (doing and being aspects, or male and female aspects) relate in harmony rather than in disharmony by asking what each needed from the other. She realized at every one of those ages, she had done it; she had accomplished or overcome the obstacle. Now she had to own her ability for herself. Throughout the process, I helped her release her survival fear at each level and to release the fears into the bonfire (which we constructed early on in the process), to help in the transformation.

Her system was further weakened by her exhaustion. Because there were so many things coming at her all at once, she contracted into old patterns that she thought she had handled. By the end of the session, she had grown up her inner children, put her adult self in charge again, rebalanced her system by opening up the lower chakras as she released the fear contraction, and she was a different person. I strongly suggested that she rest, get a massage, spend time alone (as this helps her regenerate) and don't do anything for the next 24 hours but be with herself. She took my advice and while her challenges still had to be met, she was aware that she needed more rest, even after taking some time alone, she was able to handle each situation one by one with awareness and without fear. She was able to handle them with even-temperedness and much more reasonable pacing. Subsequently, she came in over the following two weeks for additional support during this rough time of transition to keep herself balanced.

The Heart Path process is a visual and sensory process. For some this appears to be a problem. Sometimes people say to me that they are not visual. I usually say if they can tell me what they had for lunch and remember the smells and sensations, they can do this process. However some people do not 'see' as much as they may use 'smell', 'hear' or 'feel' to 'get' the aspects of self. Sometimes they feel a presence of one aspect or another. This is important, because however they get the information about themselves is how they get it. Validate it! Your job is to acknowledge what they *have* inside, rather than what they don't. If someone is very wounded, they may have developed aspects that are coping with basic functionality. For example, a child may be trying to manage the activities of the self rather than the adult, as in my last example. This is a problem, especially with those from alcoholic or drug addicted families. In order for the client to cope with a dysfunctional, unstable household, they needed to take some control themselves and be the adult prematurely. This pattern is not released unless they feel their own adult self is responsible and stable enough. Sometimes the teenager is the active one who is trying to control everything internally. Just the realization that this is so, by the observing adult client, is a revelation for them. I usually guide the client with statements such as, "Wow, no wonder it has been so hard to function! You have the child/teenager trying to cope and it isn't their job. It is the adult's job!" Then the truth of that statement resonates with them and they make a shift. We can suggest they release the fears of the child (into the bonfire) and grow that aspect up beyond childhood, or sometimes that aspect needs to play in the heart garden as a child while the adults take over and run things.

One of my most evolved students does not 'see' her aspects, instead she perceives feeling 'streams'. That is enough! That is good. Without the construct of chakras or other ways of perceiving ourselves, a stream of energy is actually more accurate. Any way that the life force energies of a person are perceived is fine. The Heart Path process gives my clients what they need as I validate their experiences. At the same time, as I perceive from my perspective and give them feedback, my observations give the client extra support. As Louise Hay says, "I listen to that internal ding to get my information." My clients learned to do same thing. Clients know what they need as they have their own internal 'ding'. We can then listen for that in our initial conversation with them to discover what they need and move into the work at hand.

Another way that I work is that I know *they* have the answers within to their healing process. This may sound redundant, but it is another aspect of *knowing* when you are on to the thread that leads to healing. Always I go with what is true for them over what I might perceive. If I perceive something different than they do, I usually let them know, but I go with what the client perceives first. The truth is you will perceive in a different visual language other than the client because you have your own life experiences. However the symbols and the story essence will be the same.

In one such case, a 44-year-old white female I will call Doris (not her real name) came in with great visual messages but she was not able to interpret them. She was looking for a "rational" or 'logical" answer. As we began Heart Path, I asked her to bring the blockage of what was stopping her from having a relationship (which was her main issue) to the front of the Heart Garden. Now we had been working on this issue in 6 previous sessions, always in combination with job related topics as well. But we had not gotten to the core issue. Often I am a few steps ahead of the person and sometimes I am *not* correct in what is the very next thing for them, but they always know. So her imagery was of a large cement block with the words "You have to do it alone" etched into the side. She was quite angry, as the message was written in a child's hand. She thought it was a mocking message from the Universe telling her that she would not have a relationship in this lifetime.

However, when I asked her to go into her feelings about the cement, she said it was cold, and felt fearful. I asked her to send the block love. As she did so, it began to melt. She saw her six year old with a crayon and she was the one who had written the message. Then I asked her to invite her six year old into the Heart Garden, and she did. When we began the dialog with the child, "You have to do it alone" was the core message that she had been given at that age by her Mother. As I questioned her further, I asked the adult if that is what her Mother really said. She reported that her mother meant to support her child in knowing herself and not giving herself up for a man. She had had this conversation with her mother, but the child still heard her own interpretation, even though she could repeat to me verbatim what the mother had actually said. "Don't give yourself up for a man." This was not what the child interpreted. "You have to do it (life) alone" was the child's interpretation. I asked the adult if she knew herself and was clear that she would not change to please a man. She said, "How could I change for him? I know myself too well." Then I asked if she believed God wanted her to be alone. Her answer was "No, I know I am suppose to have a partner. God gave me that desire!" At that the 'cement' dissolved completely, and the child was happy to throw her crayon into the fire giving up control over this issue. I asked her once again to bring any blocks to the front of the garden that prevented her from having a relationship, and nothing came, except flowers growing along the path outside her heart garden.

By following the thread of her unfolding process and taking her imagery at face value, I found that she was not seeing that she (child ego) had created the cement block not God, or the Universe. Her presence with the aspect as it *was* did the healing. She came to the understanding that now that she loved all of herself, she could love another. This was why the child had created this block, so that she would love herself first.

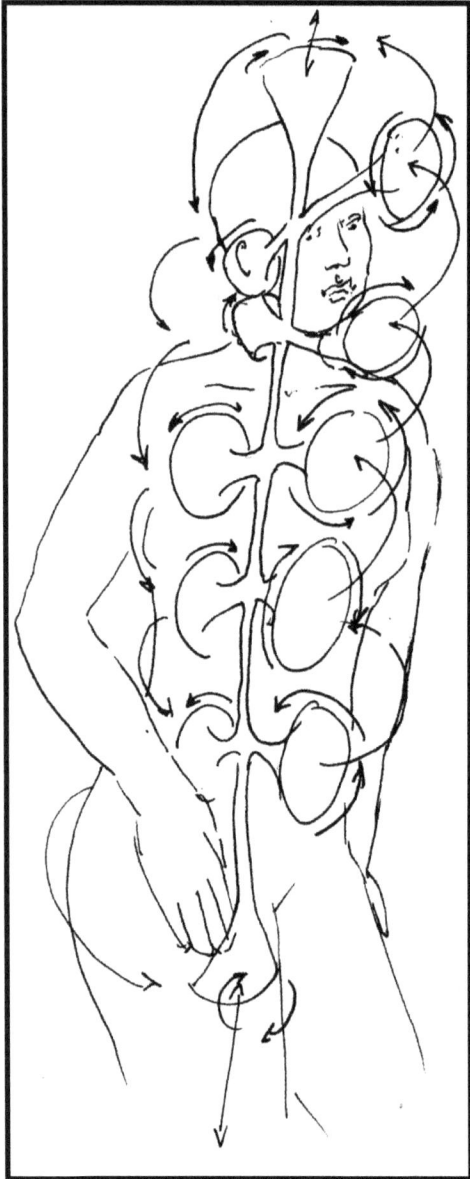

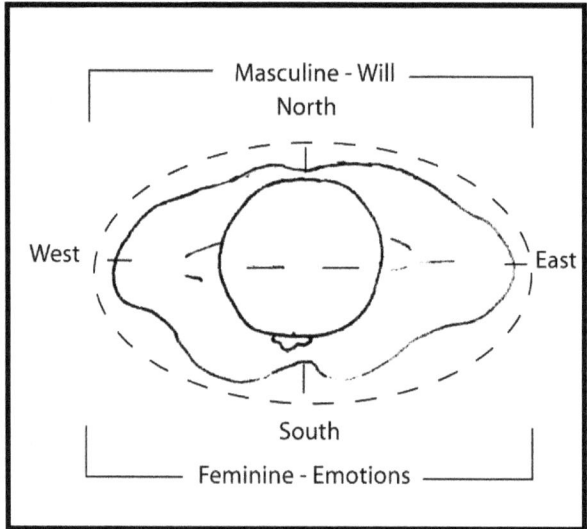

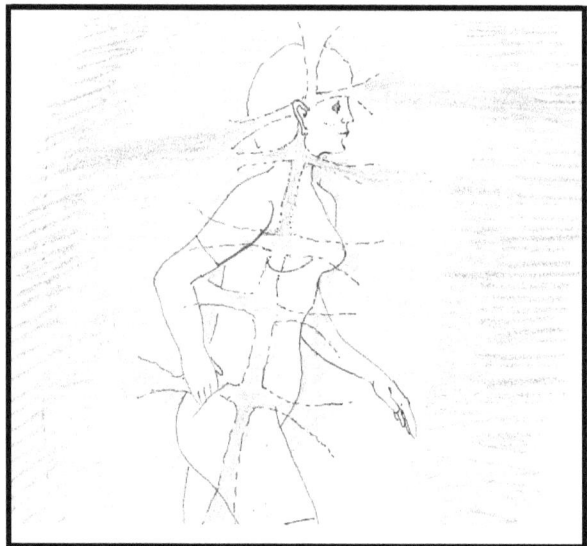

Above: Dynamics of the Human Aura from Heart Path
Top right: The human brain/body and the four directions.
Lower Right: How the field is perceived energetically.

The Brain parts as related to the Heart Path Process and their archetypes.

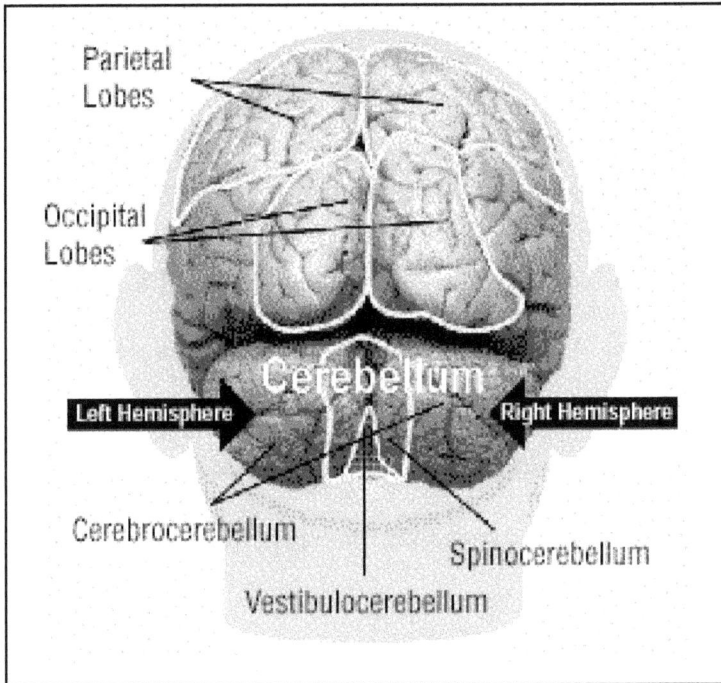

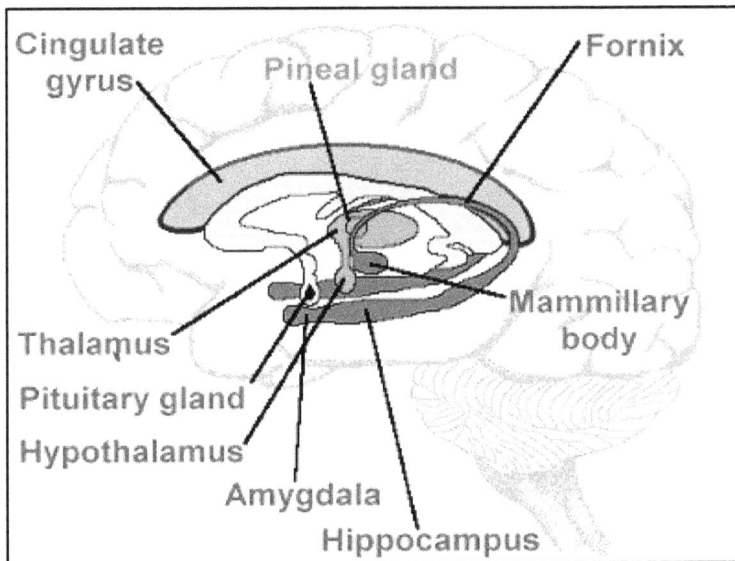

Left brain equals Doing Nature or inner male, (controls the right side)

Right brain is the Being Nature or inner feminine, (controls the left side)

Central brain or corpus callosum,

is sense perception, or Higher Self, (talks to both sides and witnesses), also houses the pineal and pituitary

glands

Back Brain Cerebellum Child

Brain Stem Animal Nature

Illustrations from the brainlabs.com

When a client loves what has been in exile, then there is reconciliation and more coherence. Their presence—with that which they have *not* been present—gives the healing. My presence with them helps them focus and helps them do the healing by containing their energy and supporting their unfolding process throughout the process of guidance that Heart Path offers. I also can suggest a different interpretation to the imagery as in the last case.

Often, they have to do the opposite of what they have been doing to right the balance. If they have been focusing on what doesn't work, we have to point to what does. If they have been focused and berating them selves for not doing what they need to, we have to acknowledge their feelings, and point out that beating themselves up does not work but love does. There may be a reason they cannot move forward that they have not viewed in themselves yet. They have a higher self; our job is to help them be aware of it. They have an inner child, inner parents, animal nature, and they often know what they are coming in for; we are just helping them see more clearly their internal dynamics and issues. We help them heal places in themselves where they can let go, forgive, transform or otherwise support a more essential expression of who they are. Of course our presence with them supports their process, and their presence with the self. The perception of the healer is significant. Often I find that during the session the client is ready for what it is I perceive. Often they want to know over their perception, but I always ask their views first. Very often I am surprised as they are by what their spirit offers up for healing. I can have an idea about what is going on, but until they go into their hearts and really look, it may not be the same as my idea. When I look at their aura, then we know a bit more, but until they go in we do not have the whole story. This is another reason to let them lead with their needs rather than imposing a mental construct of ideas or perceptions on them.

Heart Path is not a model imposed over the person. It is a process that works within and makes more conscious what is already there. I do not advocate imposing a model over anyone. Models are about thought systems, not about discovery of self. Models often confuse, and confusion becomes deeper and more difficult to release, rather than processes that guide one directly to the self. Models can be helpful if developed from observation. The problem comes when they become a standard-one-size-fits-all.

What I have found after and during the process of using Heart Path is that people love their lives more abundantly and find inner peace. They have healthier relationships, and they move more quickly along their path cutting through what they no longer need from the past. They also can view the ego in its various aspects. This allows one to love it. As we love the ego, we can begin to see that we are both primitive and enlightened at the same moment. In other words, it moves people along their path to their highest and wisest good, that of Self-Realization and Self-Love.

How to Know When To Use Heart Path

In any session that you might offer a client, there are times when Heart Path might be helpful. As you get to know the process, you will know what is needed. However, when a person seems to be at an impasse in their process, feels up against the wall, and they have circled the same issues many times, this is a perfect time! Heart Path can cut through the confusion. It is an accelerated path to healing, and it works amazingly well.

The *Heart Path* process offers first of all, a way to ground one's energy so that the client can access all of themselves. This means from their Highest Self to their Earth Self and everything in between. It helps them focus in the now, brings them ultimately into this present moment, which centers them. Then the process helps them sort the issues, as well as view themselves from an observer perspective with more compassion and elegance. It is then that the healing of the self can take place. It can open for them because they begin with their Highest Self and ground that energy, establishing the witness reality inside them. It is the witness that heals in each person through his or her distance from the drama of each person's story. This may seem like a lot for a simple meditation, however it really works for all of these things and rather quickly.

Archetypes and the Inner Self

Heart Path is based on archetypes or aspects of self that are natural extensions of our brains and our bodies. They are not merely symbolic. They are literal aspects of the self as mentioned previously. They help us understand our very nature. They help us perceive the messages that we are trying to relay and heal the wounds that are there to heal.

Again, these archetypes are primarily the Inner Child, the Animal Nature, the Inner Mother or Being Nature, Inner Father or Doing Nature, and the Higher Self. Also there are many others, teen-ager, elder, etc. However each of the main aspects mentioned correspond to the various aspects of the brain. The right and left hemispheres control the left and right sides of the body also known as receptive and extending aspects. The brain stem is the animal nature, the back brain the inner child, and the corpus callosum or the central brain that communicates with both sides of the brain and is also in communication with all of the self; the Higher Self. This is also the perceptual center of the brain where the 6th charka center ties into the pineal gland, and the crown into the pituitary gland. These glands sit right in the center of the brain.

When we engage these aspects we are also activating the chakras and helping to develop the perceptual senses.

In general the purpose of even symbolic archetypes is the same, to help us understand various aspects of our being, which in turn helps us become more conscious of who we really are in all our complexity and diversity. As mentioned previously, some psychologists and anthropologists have defined archetypes as the Queen, King, Magician, Lover, Warrior, etc. I prefer the inner family, as it is more true to where we are now, in the reality of the twenty-first century. The King and Queen archetypes may enter our inner heart garden, however their images are tied to the past of European patriarchal history and we are much more diverse than this in the present day. Also in truth, not every one can be a Queen or King in the real world in the 21st century. Most of us in the past were surfs!

The one remaining constant and common play of characters that remain real to each one of us are our families, no matter how broken. Even if a parent was absent, which is all too common these days, all of us have a mother and father in order to get to be in a body. From these archetypes we can come into a better awareness of self and realize how amazing we actually are. We can also *build* a healthier internal family than the one we may have come out of, and this in turn will help those in future generations. As we heal ourselves we heal the planet.

Deep Listening

Most of us working in a therapeutic sense are listening to something that tells us what to do next. First of all we are listening to the clients. Every nuance of what they say. This deep listening is part of any therapist's magic bag of techniques. It should be the first one for us to use in order to really hear what is being said. Deep listening is really about what is being said *under* the words. That is the emotional content. Of course we also begin with accumulated knowledge and supervision from mentors that can also help us know what to do next. Our training is crucial. Learning to know also is learning to listen to that gut feeling, it can be the 'ding' that Louise Hay refers to, that tells you what you are offering hits the mark.

On the other hand, there are divine guides that each of us have and we can receive messages from them. It can be a visceral, stereo, 'Technicolor' experience of spiritual entities filling the room giving you information for the session. Most of the time intuitive insights are like an internal 'ding'. If you are deeply listening, and get surprised by the advice, or haven't thought of it before, the guides are with you giving you that information. They give us new thoughts if we listen. They give us new ideas. Once we are in the flow of the Universe, we are directly accessing Source. Some healers naturally have this. But most of the time it has to be learned. The Navajo people call this the Dreamer, or the One Who Dreams; we are living out the dream created by the Creator to help other divine aspects of the creator come home to themselves.[6]

---

6   Duran, Ph.D., Eduardo, Buddha in Redface, Writers Club Press, NY, 2000

Since the Dream is collective, each of us can access this 'dream' through a process of grounding our energy and connecting with our higher self. Always, always, we are accessing source and guidance when we are in tune with this 'flow' of Universal information.

You might ask how would you know the information you get is from the "Highest and Wisest" source? There are several ways. The first is that in the beginning of the session you set your intention for the "Highest and Wisest Good to come to the person for the good of all beings." When you set intention, the channel opens through grounding into the center of the Earth and opening your crown chakra, then you only have to ask and wait. When information comes from our higher selves, what you get is harmless—completely harmless—information that only does the client the highest good. The information is always completely helpful information. It is fun and gentle, and enlightening and surprising. Of course you must do all of this without fear. Is that a tall order? Well, I think it all keeps us honest and humble because we cannot do it all alone. We need help and new input and that is what this book primarily offers you as a therapist: more help in your own process; connection with divine guidance; and a way to support your clients in their healing with a method that transforms consciousness.

If you do get harmful information, which is rare and does not happen, you must ask, "Who is speaking?" "Are you of the light?" If no answer comes or they do not respond, dismiss them immediately, and just let them go. You have just attracted the wrong entity. Begin again and this time set the space with gold light and proceed with your intention for the session out loud with the client, and continue as instructed above. You might also check your fear; as well to be sure you are not afraid of something within the session.

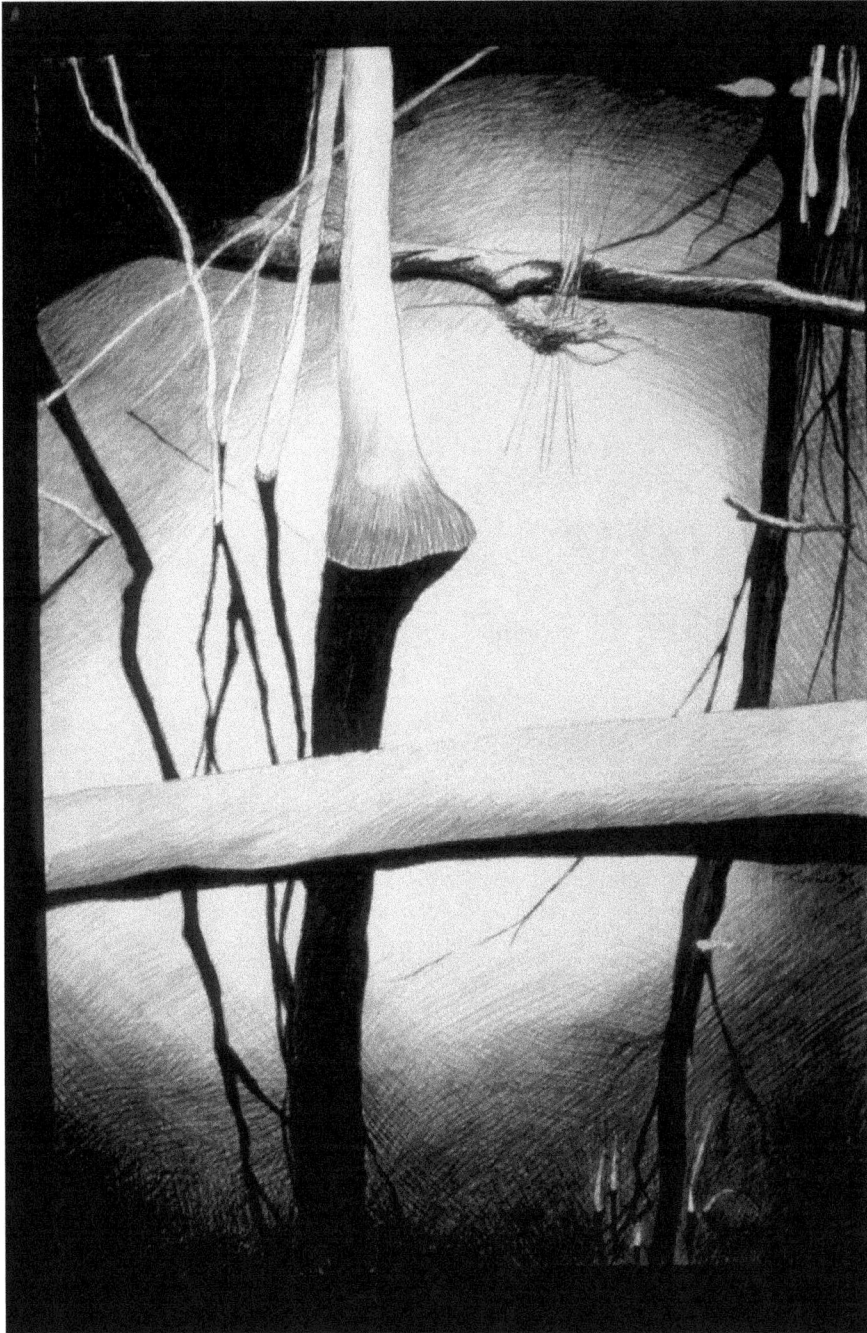

Alone Being - Charcoal on Japanese Paper
by the AUthor

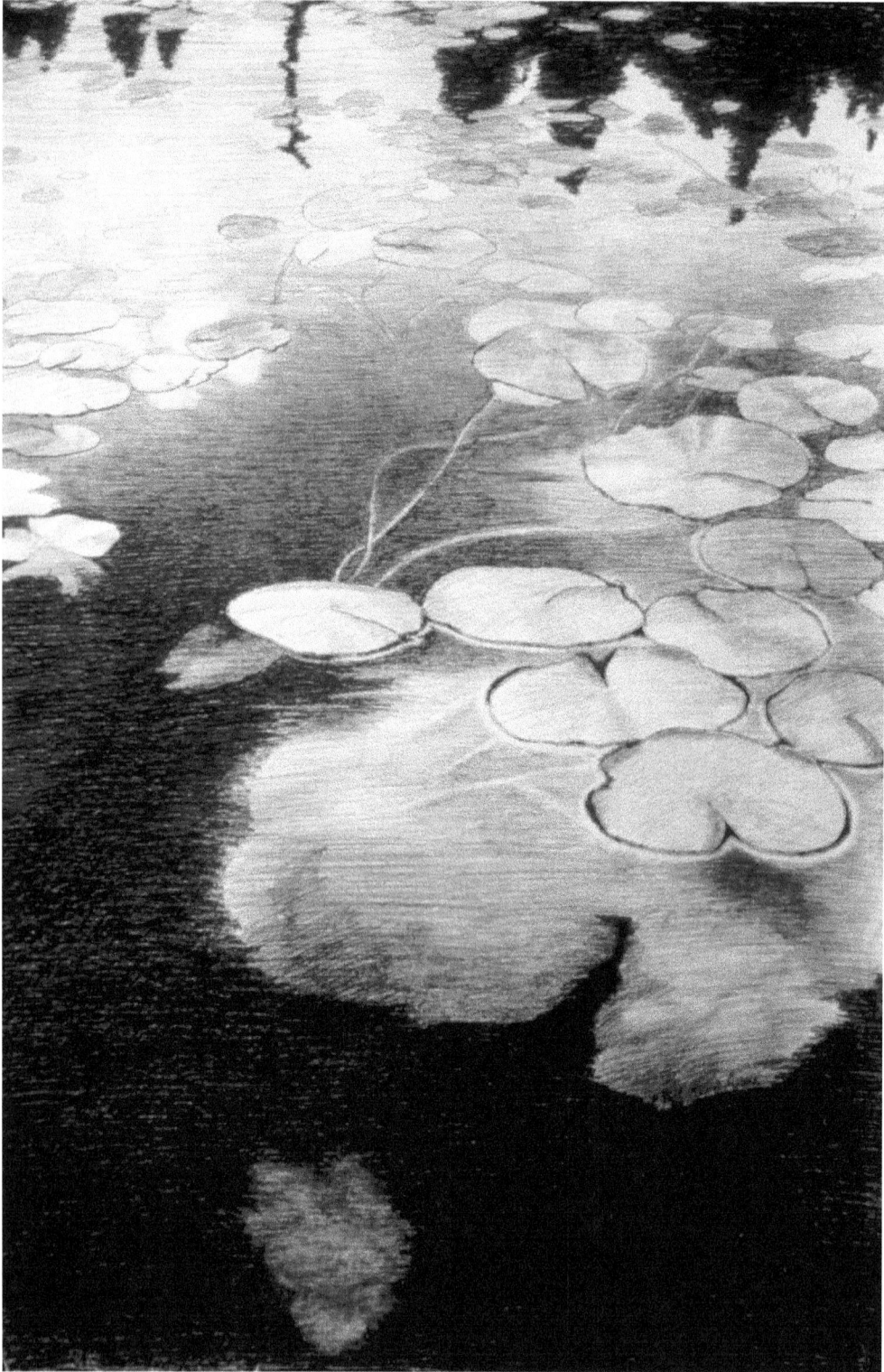

Dark and Light Reflections - Charcoal Painting
by the Author

Chapter 2 – Heart Path Meditation

<u>Harvest</u>

Sit in the garden of roses and thorns.

Take a moment to soak in your own sun.

Feel your own longing

drawing you into its fragrance.

The Universe is continually expanding.

We are the ones contracted.

This field of ripe grain

is ready for bread.

The Heart Path process works for people of any gender, race or ethnic orientation. (I will discuss gender in more detail on page 45.) In the Heart Path process, the first step is to ground the energy. The process for grounding comes from *Heart Path, Learning to Love Yourself and Listening to Your Guides,* and will give you the basic steps of the meditation. Later, I will elaborate more fully each of the steps. I have updated the meditation to my current use of it, as all things even healing processes, evolve.

Before you try this process on anyone, including yourself I suggest that you read through the entire Chapter 2 or better yet complete the book and then start again with the basic meditation. This way you will have all the necessary information before you begin. You might put the meditation on a tape for yourself, or purchase my CD that has this professionally recorded. It can help you a great deal to learn the process. Before beginning the meditation, I often check in with the person to see why they have come to see me. Once that information is obtained, and I know the basic story, I then suggest we 'set the space.'

I always connect with the light above my head drawing light through my body then connect to my grounding cord, before I begin to work with a client. The following gives you a step-by-step view of my process with clients. It helps the client immensely, so I make this my first imagery step with them as we do this together.

Grounding Meditation

I always begin any session with a circle of gold light wrapped around the client and myself. As you and the client's eyes are closed, you can use the invocation: "Drawing a circle of gold light around us, I ask for this session for my highest and wisest good and for the good of (name) my client." Setting intention is crucial for a good and positive session. Gold is used rather than white, because white light creates a polarity that sometimes attracts both negative and positive energies. Gold is neutral, and causes no polarization. It is the color of God or All-That-Is in metaphysics.[7] You are creating a deeper space in which to work. Sit in silence for a moment and visualize the gold light. Allow yourself to feel it. This color helps us move into a higher state of consciousness and gives more grounding to the work. While I am affirming this, I imagine my light grounding into the Earth and connecting with the Heart of the Earth Mother. Often at this moment, I open my eyes and check in with the client and see what is needed. If they are exhibiting challenges from being out of balance, or from having internal conflict, then I listen to them, and start the Heart Path process as indicated by what they are telling me.

Further Grounding with the Three Stars of the Self-: Begin the visualization with the star or lotus above the head. Imagine that this is connected with the higher Self (as it is). This light is from above them, shining into the head and down the neck, the arms and into the heart through the core. There is a second star or lotus in the heart center (or chakra), and now

---

7 Another way to do this mediation is to imagine for a moment that you are a tree and that from your feet you grow roots into the earth from your head grow branches. Once you imagine this, continue by breathing into the heart chakra and expanding the safety of your heart for yourself. Take five deep breaths to clear the space in the heart. If the client feel emotional pain as they focus on the heart, keep them breathing and focused on the breath using the breath as a clearing agent, and feel their feelings until they are complete with the feelings. Then with their breath, take several deep breaths, gathering your life force from the Earth; then exhale up through your body through hips, knees and feet into the heart. From Heart Path Learning to Love Yourself and Listening to Your Guides, Blue Bone Books, Santa Cruz, CA 2007.

visualize that star connecting with the first star and radiating light around your client's heart. Now move down the body to the third star or lotus, which sits in the second chakra. This is the creative and sexual center. These three stars are connecting the person with their own light primarily. Now guide them to see the light from the third pelvic star into the root and down each leg, and imagine that the three cords spiral together below the Earth to form a rope. The rope spirals down into the Earth and connects with the heart of the Earth. (I always do this within myself with my client in my own body, and it grounds me for the session as well.) If the cord rooting the client doesn't fall easily, suggest to them that they imagine that grease or a liquid like water that can energetically lubricate it. You might also remember that the Earth is magnetic, and the grounding cord naturally will be drawn into the heart of the Earth if one allows it. Bring the Earth's energy into your heart, and mix it with your heart energy by breathing several times into your heart center. Mix the energy of the Earth with the sky energy in the heart. Now the client and you are anchored in the reality of the Universe. That is how life force moves throughout our bodies, from Earth to sky and back again. You have just cleared the channels.

Core Path of the Heart Meditation-Hold the space for the client, while your client does the meditation. I watch the face very carefully to see how deep they are. If they take time to answer you, this is good, as they are in deeper space than ordinary conversation and that is where you want them to be during the guided imagery.

Say to your client: Now breathe into the heart and create a space for your self in your heart. Imagine that your breath clears away any cloudiness. Now imagine that you have a garden in your heart. It can be manicured or wild, near the water, or near the ocean. Allow it to emerge. Don't try to force it. Feel it emerge. Whatever you choose, allow what is there to be there without trying to change or manipulate the images. Take your time. Just allow the images to arise. Inside your garden notice if you have boundaries for your heart. *Is there a fence around it, or a hedge, wall, or tree circle that defines your space from others? Is the garden expansive or tiny? Pay attention to what is true of your heart. If you decide to change it, allow it to change the way you desire your safe heart-space to be. Call in the Girl Scouts or the Boy Scouts for help if you need to do heavy lifting or planting or fence building. (They can return to the heart as often as they like. Eventually living from the heart will become second nature.) It is important to know that you do not have to allow others into this space. It is yours. If they come with the respect of sacred ground then you can let them in, otherwise keep them outside of your most precious, heart garden. A boundary around the heart space is a good idea, invite the client to build or create a boundary between their heart and others for the sake of this work.

Once the garden has been created, invite into it aspects of the self who reflect the inner nature. These *archetypes* help us begin to relate to various aspects of our being, which in turn helps us become more conscious of who we really are in all our complexity and diversity.

Inner Child - Begin with the inner child. Invite the inner child into the heart garden. Notice the child that appears in the heart garden. For some it may be a long awaited reunion. Others may encounter a happy, sad, or despondent child. Do not try to control, manipulate, or direct the child's actions. Instead, just observe and notice the actions of the child and how he or she corresponds to the playful, feeling nature. You may also have more than one child, and at different ages. Greet the inner child with love. Notice how they are, agitated, skipping, happy, sad, and note how old they appear to be.

Animal Nature - When the child is there, invite in the animal nature. Notice what animal enters and notice how many animals there may be. You may have one, or many, flying, creeping, or walking creatures. It is important to note whether or not this creature is one who walks on the earth or swims in the sea. If it is a creature of the sea, such as a whale or dolphin, you might also invite in a four-legged animal, as they teach us how to walk on the Earth. Sea creatures know about feelings and swimming through the waters. Both are helpful. But the Earth ones are more helpful in a body.

Inner Feminine or Being Nature Next, when you are ready, invite in the inner-feminine nature. This is the *being* aspect of our nature. She may be represented by a mother image; a feminine image of one's self, or someone known to the client. Whether a person is male or female, they have an inner *being* nature. Allow the image of your inner being nature to take shape. If you visualize an image of your actual mother, have the aspect of you step out of the image of your mother. Let the birth mother go out of the heart garden. The image of your feminine will remain. The inner feminine is not the actual birth mother, or adopted mother, but the woman inside one's self.[8] It does not matter if you are male or female; you have a feminine consciousness. Invite her in and see how she relates to the other aspects of the self. Does she know the child and the animal? Is she familiar with your heart garden? What does she look like? She is the "being" part of one's nature. Just allow her to be who she is. If you have trouble visualizing her, do not worry, just make a space for her and keep going; at some point she will arrive. If you have trouble visualizing a woman, just invite in your being nature, the aspect that is able to *be with* yourself or others. (The client may need to grow into 'being'. Sometimes the aspect will not appear right away. Just make a space for it and it will most likely show up later.) Be sure to leave a space of silence for your client to have his or her own process in each of these visualizations. Encourage them to feel each one entering.

Inner Masculine or Doing Nature - Next, call in your inner masculine aspect. This is the male aspect of your being—the one who knows about going out into the world and who also knows how to live in the world. It may be felt as a *doing* aspect not related to sex. He is the protective side of our beings that can also be playful and responsible— the *doing* aspect of who we are in the world. This masculine aspect can manifest in our heart gardens as brother, father and/ or a busy doing aspect of our own form. This is not your actual birth father. This is your *inner* father/brother/doing aspect of you. For some, the inner male may be a challenge to bring in,

---

8   Often people will begin using internal images of other people they admire, or those who have had great influence on them such as Hollywood stars, or their mother or grandmother's image. These are often there to guide a person into a sense of self. This is fine, however for the client to know *themselves* they need to replace this image with one of themselves. When they are ready to do this they will tell you. You can always ask them if they need to keep or release the image of another.

especially men or women with abusive pasts from their birth father or a male close to the family in the father role. Just know that your inner father does not have to be abusive. He can be nurturing, loving and kind, as well as action oriented. As your inner feminine may not be perfectly clear right away, do not feel you have to bring the inner father in right away either. Just make the space for him to show up. Do not be disturbed if he does not come right away. He will come when the rest of the family feels safe enough or when, you or the client, are ready. Often there is something that needs to be established beforehand if the inner father is not coming in. It may be a sign that abuse has happened, and the rest of the inner child, inner feminine, or both are not willing to have them there. It may be that these aspects are abusive to themselves or punishing this aspect for the sins of the father. If you ask the client to make a space, then the safety can be established internally and they will often spontaneously 'pop' in later. Trust of the self is what needs to be established first, and sometimes that takes time.

Higher Self or Observer Nature- Next invite in your higher self, your all-wise, all-knowing self. This aspect holds much of the wisdom of life and can be asked what to do when visionary wisdom is required. This aspect may appear as light, or as a God/Goddess Divine figure. It may appear to the client as an angel or being of light, it could be very ethereal or it could be more like a Mother Nature Goddess aspect. Notice interactions between all the aspects and how they relate together. Ask your client to describe each of the aspects of the self. This will tell you a great deal about their perceptions of the self and how they see themselves.

Listen closely to what is showing up. Again, this is not to be manufactured through the mind, but allowed to emerge through a heart-felt opening. All through the meditation I would suggest you (as the Therapist) pay attention to what arises for you as you read through the meditation. Notice your own heart garden and which aspect shows up and which ones don't. If not all the aspects are present this may indicate several things. It could be an aspect you are working on or developing. It could be that an aspect is being blocked by emotions, such as fear, grief or anger. Just be with the feelings and yourself and don't try to make it different. Just notice.

One client I have had was preoccupied by guilt from divorcing her former husband and wasn't able to be present to herself as a result. She blamed herself for his decline. All she saw in the heart was her relationship with him, and her sadness. When we worked through and processed the guilt, her inner masculine and feminine were able to "show up". Check to see if there are emotions that are running rampant and need to be cleared first either with your client or yourself. Another client had a higher self in an executive business suit. She came to the conclusion that this was not her true higher self but a part of her that thinks it is in charge. We just observed it and witnessed its interactions with the other aspects of self. Very often the client will "see" what is going on inside them and willingly shift to a more authentic identity.

Other Aspects of the Self -While these five are the primary aspects, you may notice that your client has others come to the heart garden such as the teenager, one's self at present age to be the referee or the observer, or a distinctive observer aspect, or these may spontaneously be there inside themselves without prompting. The teenager often holds the truth of an emotional state frozen in time from those difficult years. Sometimes this aspect is exhibited in the client's behavior if you listen closely. I often watch the person and feed back what I am hearing about them from them. When I ask how old that aspect is, they often know the age. Then a memory often comes in from that age where the client is holding memories, a belief or thought that they have not worked through. If I ask, what happened at 10 or 6, they usually remember. Then I offer what I perceive in their field. I notice if I perceive a child, teenager, or adult, arriving and ask if they are aware that there is a part of them that is not happy and needs to speak up. Sometimes they are not aware, and it gives the opportunity to use this Heart Path process to discover the aspect for them selves. Again this might be where I would let them lead, unless they are stuck in the process and don't know where to go next.

Certain ages depicted to the client, (Adolescent, age 7, 8, 3, 9 or any other specific age) gives you much information. The age of their inner child or adult that presents itself matters tremendously. The inner child comes in most frequently between the ages of 4-6. This is the age when most children are in the playful mode and have most fun. Of course this is not always true if there has been any sort of trauma during the youth of the client. However, when the child comes in at another age, say 9 or 1 this is an indication that something happened at that age. The child is presenting the age where the trauma occurred. It doesn't have to be abuse; it could be a loss, a time when they were scared or when they had a change in their environment.

A question such as: "What do you remember about that age?" or "Did anything happen at that age that comes to mind?" Your questions can support them to remember, to re-member their coherence. Depending on the client, a more open-ended question, such as the first one suggested, might be more effective.

If they give you an indication of trauma, I always remind them that "that was then and this is now" and ask if they would like to release the emotion around that incident. If they do, then I ask them to create a fire in the heart garden and see if they can release the pain into the fire. (I will discuss the bonfire in a later section).

If the aspect is a teenager however, there is certainly more life changing issues or challenges or decisions that likely occurred at that age. *How* it matters is to be determined by questions put to the client about that time in their lives. In working the Heart Path process, the story is useful in order to perceive what decisions, beliefs or trajectories the client has made at that time in their lives that may no longer be useful for them. Dissolving unnecessary belief systems is the key to helping the person transform. I perceive an unnecessary belief much like a pulled thread in fabric. It restricts freedom and flow, and is not useful if it is hurting the full movement of the fabric of the individual.

More on The Inner Child – So much work has been done with people in psychology investigating and attending to the Inner Child. In R.C. Swartz book, *Internal Family Systems Therapy*[9], the wounded inner child is called an "exile." That is because the psyche is trying to defend against the pain the child felt in the past. They exile the aspect into unconsciousness

---

9   R.C. Swartz, *Internal Family Systems Therapy,* Guilford Press, NY, 1995 pg. 231

in order to protect their conscious selves from feeling the pain. However, in the Heart Path process, they can reunite with those aspects and become more conscious and whole. Releasing tears is healing for the client. Let them cry and move on when they complete the wave of grief.

Often in traditional therapy, the child is taken into consideration, but not always taken into consideration *in relationship with the other aspects of the inner family*. This is one way Heart Path differs from other ways of working with clients. The whole inner family is called forth in relation to the child aspects, as well as to each other. This creates a fuller picture of the dynamics of the inner world and brings them to consciousness. Before one can shift a toxic dynamic, one must see it. Once it is seen, or brought to awareness, the shifting begins to happen by just shedding light on the issue at hand.

The needs of the children are important just as any child's needs are important. Infants are to be loved cradled and held and attended to as any mother or father will tell you. So the inner parents are there to watch over them. When a child reaches two to three the child is here to play and enjoy their childhood until seven years old when pre-pubescences sets in. Their play might be geared to more adult concerns at that time. At eight to twelve they are entering adolescence, or pre-adolescents, they are experimenting with being an adult. This is another stage altogether and a very important one. The pre-adolescent (8-12) makes the first attempts to experiment with adulthood. Sometimes great changes can occur for the child; school changes occur, new siblings are born, their parents sometimes divorce or have divorced. All of it sets the stage for the child's experiences of moving into adulthood. Anyone going through transitions in their adult life will relive adolescent patterns set during this beginning period in adolescents. The client is often unconscious of the wound until that child aspect at that age appears again in meditation. What matters is what shows up. That is what you can work with in the session. Again, asking the right questions of that aspect contributes to the healing. There will be a section on questions later in this chapter.

Children cannot and should not run the parental energies to work and make a way through any adult life. The adults need to be in charge, kids need to play. Often when we are hurting, scared, out of work, or in transition, the clients will find themselves with a child part that is reliving some trauma from youth. They get scared and take over. It is up to our adult selves to put their arms around the child and hold them, while the adults navigate the situation. The adults know how, the child must follow, or the child will run into trouble and all kinds of illness issues forth. Often when in a crisis, we let the emotions of the child get us tied up in knots instead of letting the adults calm us and take over. I find this almost every week in many clients. So it is something to look out for with your clients. Often times, if a child had an alcoholic parent or an absent parent and had to act as the parent for the other siblings or had to take care of the incapacitated parent, the child takes over in situations that are similar, as the person will have that pattern still operating from childhood. As the person grows up, sometimes the child is still running things internally as a false adult. Heart Path allows them to be 'arrested' so that they stop. It helps people grow up emotionally. Often when a child is running things, it helps to let them know that their belief "I have to take care of things myself' is not working anymore. This allows them to stop. They can come into the heart garden and throw it into a campfire[10], and then agree to release control. The adult may have to say something like; 'Don't worry, I am here to take charge, it is my job.' Sometimes the child has never had a chance to play. Once the child releases control, and the adult takes over, the child is free to play, and the adult knows what needs to happen next. Often externally the adult needs to cut loose, and sometimes there is a period of time where the adult is catching up on play. You could call it delayed adolescence or you could say it is simply a rebalancing of the internal dynamics. You see this with many adults in mid-life crisis.

Some readers of this last imagery may feel I am prescribing behavior on the inner family. This is not the case. I have discovered that there is inherent sense of justice that the inner world holds; the children need to be cared for by parents, and not the other way around. The adults need to take responsibility for the life being lived, and the higher self or

10   See page 42.

the observer nature is there to love it all. As we feel into these aspects, the moral imperative of our 'operating system' becomes obvious. This is an observation I have made that transcends race, religion or ethnic background.

A Note on Genders: Whether a client is heterosexual or homosexual or as some would say, 'otherly gendered' Heart Path can work for everybody. However, a client that is homosexual may perceive things differently. If they are truly homosexual that is they were born to love the same sex, the person's inner self will be one sex or the other, or sometimes a combination where the two 'polarities' are expressed as no gender or one gender, either male or female. For example many lesbian clients have two women inside themselves, one more masculine (doing) and one more feminine (being). Women, especially those with a history of abuse, may have one sex (female or male depending on the gender of the abuser) with whom they cannot tolerate contact. Sometimes when they have done enough healing on themselves, the offending gender will return in themselves, but not always. The same holds true for men who are homosexual. Two men will appear; one more in tune with being and one the 'doer.'

Some heterosexual men, especially if they are homophobic, cannot tolerate that they might have an inner feminine. So I often refer to the energies present, as the 'doing' (masculine) and 'being' (feminine) aspects of the self. Everyone has some form of masculine and feminine to them, or doing and being, even if it shows up as one gender only. Sometimes the person will have just one adult self with no masculine or feminine. In my work, what matters is that they are looking at themselves and paying attention to what is true for them. It is from 'what is' that a person can begin to grow. I will discuss more about the masculine and feminine later, but for now what I see about health and wholeness is that in Western Culture what often throws people out of balance is the relentless pursuit of getting stuff, which drives the male aspect into dominance and throws the system out of balance. Women as well as men have this problem. Most women don't know their femininity at all, nor the power of softness in discussing issues rather than resorting to the male aspects that want to fight.

we ascend we can see our light as the ultimate goal of identity. Often people will have more than one, and sometimes a whole zoo.[11] Each of us has an animal nature. Many people have multiple animals, whether winged, crawling or four-legged. When we get to know them, it helps us learn how we will react in a tight situation, and what we have at our disposal when we need it. Often, the cats, lions, tigers and bears, eagles or beavers, mice, snakes or lizards or whatever is contained in our menagerie are how we act or react on instinct. If one is feeling under attack, the animal will come to the foreground. It is also good to know that we have a whole cadre of critters to help us instinctually.

Often displaying or 'calling in' our animal nature will help us in a tight situation, and I have often used my animals for protection on dark streets late at night or in the city in broad daylight. They work for us, if we allow them to.

If people you work with have more than one animal nature, they have a variety that may work at different chakra levels. There are also people who use the animal nature to help themselves to greater understanding with various chakras. WuLan has something to add here, and this was from a class on the Animal Nature where I channeled WuLan.

*Animals see and sense energy instinctually. You know that dogs see energy. They see spirits and sometimes they react to them, as cats can. Cats know about energy presences. When Robin had her pet cat Minka, Minka would sit during sessions, and pay attention to what was going on energetically with the client and between the client and the space around them. The cat was watching all the time what was happening energetically. Barking dogs sometimes notice the guides coming in. So if you notice the animals in your life getting energized when you ask for spiritual guidance don't be surprised. *

Underneath the animal nature, is the primitive self. This aspect is sometimes seen as a creature with teeth; sometimes the creature is blind or deaf or has no identity. It might have

---

11   To understand what various animals offer the client, I refer often to Animal Cards, by Jamie Sams, David Carson, Angela C. Werneke, which gives in depth understanding of various animals. Also I refer to books on animals that are in the library which give us their basic instinctual behavior and how they move in and through their environment. Children's books on animals for young adolescents are especially useful, as they boil down behavior quite succinctly.

Health is a rebalance, movement out and movement inside and awareness of 'what is'. In energy work of any kind, balance is the key to health and wholeness, not getting more stuff.

Initial Key Questions to Ask Your Client: Some good questions to ask your client during the session are: 1) How do you perceive your aspects (specifically: heart garden, inner child, parents, animals, or higher self). 2) How are they getting along? 3) What are they doing/being? Or 4) How do they appear to you? 5) Does the child, parent, or animal need anything? 6) What do they want to tell you? 7) Are they all getting along with each other? Some of these questions will become obvious to ask. Once the belief is released, new agreements can be made such as; We agree to work together; I (child) agree to let the adults run the show; I (adult) will keep the child safe at all times; I (child) will tell the adult when I am not feeling safe, etc.

When a child shows up that is not the initial inner child but an aspect that comes in for healing, there are some important questions to ask the client at that point. The first is how old is the child? The second is: Is there anything that happened at that age that you recall? What beliefs did they form at that age? Or Are there any beliefs that the child acquired at that time?

More on The Animal Nature

> *The animal nature is a particular interesting aspect, which has to do with our protective nature as a result of living in a body. I mention this because our animal nature is thought to be of a lower order. This is simply not true. This is a misperception that some religious teachings have given. The animal nature is part of who we are as much as any other aspect. It moves from instinct, from being in the moment, and it offers great teaching if we allow ourselves to listen."*

Observing the animal nature is a wonderful way to get to know our basic protective instincts. If we see animal nature as a foundational element in our human structure, then we can see it as part of our wholeness, rather than dismissing animals as of a lower order. As a tail or paws or just be teeth. This lies deep within the self under feelings of inadequacy, a lost or abandon child self, or a primal part of the self connected to our survival instincts. This self can create a false self that impacts us by "shinning" in our aura without content. When we identify it, it is helpful to be with it, and feed it, bring it into the heart, and allow it to be as it is anyway. This aspect dissolves eventually, or it stays "cozy" within the heart. Allow it to be and it will help you release the false ego pattern of separation at a very deep level. Sometimes you have to hang out with it in the heart for a long time before it shifts. This could be days, weeks, or years. But keeping it in your awareness as a polar opposite of the Self, gives awareness to the depth and breadth of our being. All of us have this, by the way as the root of separation.

More About The Inner Masculine and Feminine

Pay special attention to the 'inner parents' represented by the masculine and feminine aspects of your client and how they might respond to the child. When a client is unaware of the inner "father and mother' I often find most of the problems with the relationship between these two male/female aspects. Remember that they are the 'doing' and 'being' aspects of the person. Sometimes self judges the self and this does not help relating. Do they know each other (child, and inner masculine and feminine)? Do they even like each other?

Often the inner masculine and feminine are reflected in the issues of the marriage if the client is married or in a relationship, sometimes of the client's parents. They show plainly the client's relationship with doing and being aspects of themselves. Often these two are in conflict, as they do not always work together. It may not be an exact duplicate of marital issues, but the underlying issues will be the same whether internal mates or external. When the client changes his or her inner relating, the outer often rights its self.

One example of this was a 43-year-old Latina woman who came in with a complaint of a block in her system. She felt stuck in her marriage, in her life, and out of alignment within herself. She had just broken up with her partner of several years. When we checked inside to view her inner masculine and feminine, they were not on speaking terms. They needed to begin to "make up and relate." After discovering that what they both wanted was more love and less judgment from the other, they could reconnect. They threw the judgments into the fire, and embraced.

Often I spend the first part of an initial session with the client working on this internal relationship. If the aspects love each other and have internal harmony, then they can move on to more healing of other fragmented parts. If not, and they dislike each other and have mistrust, then they need to work it out with the inner family first. Often my questioning works from "what does the inner feminine (being), or the inner masculine (doing) need from the other?" Working one at a time they take turns and speak to the other aspect. I often start with the feminine because her voice is often heard less. When they take turns and learn from the other, what is *actually* needed instead of what was thought to be needed, the dynamics shift naturally and they can begin to learn to trust each other. Remember that a sound relationship is built on the foundation of love, trust, respect, and great communication.[12] Usually one of these building blocks is missing and need to be re-established. If one or more are missing, some work on the inner family dynamics is in order. If several of them are non-existent or in need of consideration, this can also be revealed when one works with the inner self. It is often valuable to teach clients these fundamental ways in relating. Great healing can take place when we simply drop judgment of ourselves and appreciate who we are.

One of my favorite techniques is to pass a talking stick inside around the 'camp fire.' A talking stick comes from a Native American reconciliation ritual. It is a designated and often decorated stick, bowl or other such implement used for better communication. When passed from aspect to aspect, each aspect holding the stick, or bowl must speak from the heart. The other aspects are required to listen. Each aspect receives the stick or bowl when it is their turn and the shift takes place through deep listening and receiving of the true feelings

---

12   This information on healthy relating comes from Arch Angel Michael, who helped me early on find a relationship. I was asking out of much frustration, "What makes a good relationship!" and the answer came through like a thunderbolt.

by other aspects. This works wonders. By the time they have all been heard, there is usually some kind of reconciliation already occurring. If you can ask if they agree to work on trust, or communication, or respect, they can usually work on it together and have already begun to work together to transform the internal dynamics.

More About The Higher Self or Observer

The observer, or Higher Self, watches the other aspects interact. It brings unconditional love and no judgment to their interactions and to witness. The client's Higher Self, along with the other aspects, can help to integrate what is not working among the other aspects. This is especially important when there is inner conflict. Sometimes I ask the client to bring in the Higher Self and have it wrap its arms around the whole family. This helps self-acceptance and neutralizes conflict. For now, observe each aspect's interaction and see how everyone gets along.

You can also ask your client's inner Earth Mother or Earth Father to enter their heart garden. They are especially good at helping us understand our Earth-based reality, such as money, jobs, and housing and the practical things of life.

Initially all you need to do is have your client breathe and be with their inner aspects. Often there is a lot going on for them internally that they may or may not share with you. Watch their eyelids, this way you know how active the visuals are for them. You will also notice their internal dialog going on by their silence. Asking questions at this point is not helpful. However, you can ask how things are going every once in a while. Notice the interactions of their inner reality and see how their inner family is getting along. When they are ready to bring their awareness back into the room have them take five deep breaths and come back slowly, taking all the time they need. You might ask what happened for them, or if you are intuitive, you can follow along with the energetic shifts.

Multiple Aspects

Be aware that there may be more than one of each aspect. There may be two or three feminine aspects or several children or a variety of very different aspects of our inner male. This is quite common, as each aspect can hold a different awareness, can maintain very different views of reality, and can give us different views of issues until the time we are ready to integrate or change those views. Multiple aspects give us time to learn from these various aspects. They can also point out a wound from the past that needs to be healed.

In one case I had a client who had sixteen different adult aspects that were all in relationship with one another and in opposition to each other just with the male and female aspects! While it was a lot to integrate, the client was acknowledging *all* of the self.

In another example, if we have several inner children, each one may hold a belief or trauma that needs to be experienced again in order to be brought to our full awareness before the trauma can be released. The client does not always need to re-experience trauma to heal it. However, the *wound* left from the trauma does need to be acknowledged. As the client sits with the wound—and becomes compassionate towards the child—the wound heals.

Once the lesson is learned or the wound healed, the child can blend with other children or grow into a parent if it is right for the client to have this occur. This can take place by inviting the child to grow into adulthood or by having the child who has healed step into the one who has been waiting for the change to occur. This way you can help them to grow up when and if it feels right for the client. I always give them the option, and see what they want to do. Sometimes the wounded child, now healed again, needs to play awhile. Sometimes I start with the youngest wounded child and grow the child into the next age, say an 8 year old into a 10 year old, and so on. They may always have a 5-6 year old representing the inner child as a happy carefree child.

In the heart garden, the playing field is more level. The heart brings all of those aspects together in an equal way. There is no hierarchy of upper and lower. Everything is part of the divine, every aspect. This is key to bringing the self together as Self. And whether it comes as a disheveled little child who needs help, or whether it comes as an animal, which could be a bear or a coyote, or as primal elements of the animal instinctual nature, or whether it comes as an Native American or East Indian, or a tribal person or other aspect that seems different than our own reality in this life time, they all have their messages and they all have their teachings, and each is here to help us evolve. Whatever occurs in the heart garden is what the person needs to receive. I have learned to trust this implicitly.

More on the Three Stars of the Self

Many ancient traditions focus on three aspects of self, such as in the Huna tradition in Hawaii.[13] Star Woman speaks of the three stars that relate to the three levels of self in this and other traditions. The first is the head or the crown, known in Hindu philosophy as the 6th and 7th chakras. The next level of the self is the heart, or the 4th chakra, which is where all the various aspects of self come together, and the last level is in the Dantien or the 2nd chakra which is the seat of creativity, money and sense of foundation.

Here is what Star Woman said in one of my classes about the Three Stars of the Self.

"I want to speak to you about the significance of your three stars and why they are so important. The first star is about our relationship to the father, or the light, this interpenetrates all aspects of your being. The second star is about our relationship to others, to all people, friends and relations including the trees, rocks and hills, to the starfish and the sea lions, the butterfly and the muskrat. The third star relates to our foundation, that relationship to the Mother Earth, the dark, fecund living Earth. You need a new relationship to the Earth Mother because what we have had has been from the wound of mother, not the heart and reality of Mother Earth.

13   King, Ph.D., Serge Kahili, *Huna, Ancient Hawaiian Secrets for Modern Living*, Atria Books, Simon and Schuster, 2008.

"Another way to view this is this, 1/3 of your relationship is to the Earth Mother, 1/3 to those on the planet, the humans, tree people rocks and so on, The other 1/3 is with light or Spirit. They are all you; they are the entire Divine.

Now as you become aware of this, you can begin to see that what is most important is right relationship, since relating to the Earth, to others and yourself, and to the Sky is everything. If you have proper relationships to all that is, you do not need to become frantic, scared of survival, or desperate. You know that you will be provided for."

Reinventing our Relationship with the Earth-New Mother / Ancient Mother

(Star Woman continued)

"The redesigning of the Mother Earth relationship must begin with clearing the relationship with your present birth mother. Everyone has a birth mother. If your birth mother or adoptive mother as the case may be could not own up to their likeness to the all-giving and generous Earth, or b) could not transfer to you as an adult that your Mother Earth is your true mothering and nurturing self, then you could have an improper or challenging relationship to or with Earth.

"So reinventing your Mother relationship which is 1/3 of your relating to all life; is very critical at this time in history. You must begin to see that you live on a planet that gives you everything you need to live, she gives shelter, clothing, food, medicine, she gives water, herbs, rain for renewal.

"As a mother, (each woman is a mother, by the way whether they have children or not) as a mother, each woman must see their giving and caring qualities. A true mother gives everything without limits, yet, in human terms, instead of gratitude and respect for what has been given, an entitled attitude or an attitude of taking without thanks does not encourage more abundance. Instead this entitled "I deserve to have" or "I will take" without gratitude restricts the flow of generosity. No one or no reality gives with abandon to one who holds this entitled attitude.

"The paradox is that you *are* entitled. You do deserve to thrive and survive by the very nature of being. You are a divine being. You have a right to exist. That knowledge of being divine is humbling, because you know ALL of life is divine. Why would you want to hurt another?

"However if you do not know this vital piece of information, then it evokes resentment because you are not aware that you are who you are and being divine, you are loved and blessed. An attitude of entitlement cannot develop if you truly know this reality. Entitlement stems from the lack of knowing your divinity, as PART of All-That-Is rather than as a uniquely divine being.

"And as one gives gratitude you express that understanding of your divinity and claim your very birth right of being, in saying thank you to the Earth Mother, and Sky Father, you affirm and witness the miracle of your life, the miracle of your being, as you stand in THAT miracle. When you offer thanks for the simplest things, your shower, the breakfast eggs you fried, the car you own, the legs that take you for walks, you begin to feel that gratitude for the first mother, the Mother Earth. She is here for you in all her splendor, and one must be tuned into being, not the doing of it but the miracle that is your birthright.

"When you reinvent or redesign your relationship with Mother Earth you are saying thank you too for your human mother who did what she could despite the circumstances of her perceived wounds and limitations. You are saying thank you to the miracle of life giving you the opportunity to be living this life in this miracle of a planet.

"When you reinvent your relationship to your Mother Earth or birth mother, try to say thank you and acknowledge what you have received. *Thank you*, just that, and then *be* with that relationship. Be with all of your aspects of relationship with gratitude and see how you recover your humanity."

Walking In Gratitude Exercise: Try taking a walk daily for two weeks, and simply say thank you as you lay down each step. Thank you, step. Thank you, step, and just see how your life changes.

In walking this morning, I found myself drifting from the practice. My mind was wandered all over the place, thank you; thank – left step, you – right step, thank you, then I would drift again. But as I really practiced, I found myself feeling so grateful, and so much in favor of my life. Thank you for that flower, thank you for that rock, thank you for the clouds. I could also feel my liver say no, I could feel the imbedded, stubborn parts of myself say no! I could feel them unhappily making this declaration of resentment. So I noticed them and said thank you for the voices of despair and resentment, and soon they were howling with me, howling with me like wolves or coyotes, thank you, thank you. I am in love with this life!

Beyond Archetypes- Expressing our Elements of Nature

The various aspects of nature, Earth, Air, Fire and Water, and in the Chinese systems, the fifth element of metal, are part of many spiritual traditions around the world. They are called Orixas in Africa and Brazil, they are called the four directions on the medicine wheel in many Native American cultures in North and South America, as well as in Tibet, Norway and Scandinavia, with the Sami people and in other regions around the world. These traditions or spiritual paths are focused on nature *as* us. The medicine wheel, or the circle with an equidistant cross, contains a mini-version of the Earth with the four directions, Earth, Sky and the Heart, which is the center of all things. In most Native Spirituality, this symbol is the basis of all ceremonies from Sundance to Sacred Sweat Lodges.

The understanding of this is very important for our contemporary society, because we are so out of touch with nature. We have created a separate reality outside of nature in our cities and towns, houses and places of business. It is basic reason for our feelings of separation from the Earth Mother, and a foundation of human insecurity. Since man has walked up right, this has been a challenge. The late Joseph Campbell, renown story teller and professor of History at Sara Lawrence University, spoke of this often in his books and later in the television series called: The Hero's Journey, with Bill Moyers, where he described the challenges of the human journey through mythology. He was well versed in world mythology and stories and how they shape human consciousness.

Discovering Native American and African spiritualities has opened up an incredible world of awareness for me of how we are actually integrally a part of nature. It is outside of western cultural constructs so it is not easy to explain to western minds. However, each of us, no matter where we come from or who we are, expresses ourselves as a part of nature through the elements. Actually each of us *is* an element in our essential nature. That is called our Orixá in African and Brazilian theologies. We can be a combination, such as air and water in various forms, but basically we are an element of Earth, Air, Fire or Water. We are who we are at the core, and knowing the various Orixás helps us to be ourselves without guilt or shame. They indicate our basic nature without having to compromise. These are the aspects of us that do not change. They speak to us of our uniqueness, and at the same time help us become all we can be. As a poet and artist, when I understood my Orixás, and I am still comprehending them, it became clear that my path was to create. Naṇá the spring, is about two things, unconditional love and the first watery indications to feed the people what they need with clear emotions. She is the Orixá that comes up through the rocks, so my other Orixá is the rock, or Xângo (Chango), or manifested fire. This gives me the impetus to keep focused in creating. It also helps in the healing work I do, as these Orixás help in supporting those who need emotional release and clarity.

A friend of mine is an Ogum. Ogum is the second element of fire, and one of movement that exists in any of the elements as a force. No doubt, the force and speed at which he lives tells me this, his need for constant movement is primary. At sixty-one, he is a cross-country bicycler, professor, and author. He travels widely to read his work, and to teach as well as maintaining a full-time job. His need for constant adventure is clear to me. He is a river of movement in his very being, and he is not necessarily a type 'A'.

Another person with whom I am familiar has the Orixá Ossáe. Ossáe is the wounded healer who is totally into healing herbs and the properties of healing through plants. Her interest in herbs and medicines from plants preceded her initiation, and it was quite wonderful to have it confirmed and witnessed by a group of us in Brazil. Her initiation confirmed who she was in a more public way. Orixá initiations tend to affirm who one is rather than invalidate or diminish who one is.

Traditionally to find out your Orixá the process involves initiation and divining rather than a rationally thought process of thinking about which one might be us. In Comdomblé and Umbanda, which I studied in Brazil in Temple Guaracy, the Orixá of any individual was discovered through ceremony. It was not a process that one could duplicate in this country very easily as it takes a group with the right songs and the right intentions. In Umbanda, one receives their Orixá after a long process with a spiritual guide (or Angel) called a Kaboklo. The Kaboklo helps you find your Orixá. Some people take years to discover who they are, while others find it quickly.

In Condomblé one's Orixá comes first and then you take time after the initiation to learn about what just happened! Watching a person find their Orixá in Condomblé looks as though the person is falling asleep, but they are not falling asleep, they are being drawn out of hiding! Actually, they are receiving the element that matches their inner essence. They are emerging from the illusion of who they thought they were into an alignment with who they actually are in their essence.

Exercise: Whose Eyes Are You Looking Through?

Once you have identified the various archetypes, try looking through the eyes of each one. Start with the child, and move through the animals, feminine, masculine and higher self. Another way to do this is to begin to identify which aspect you identify with most. Whose eyes do you see through most of the time? Then write what it sees and how it thinks. Then move to the next and the next. Do not forget the higher self. This makes a huge difference when you realize that the higher self is the observer who witnesses our lives in love. When one is in the witness-self there is a more clear view of your life, and one is less tied into the emotions.

When I first tried this, it became a way to view myself. This perspective has helped me ever since to create my life from the witness state. It has helped me evolve.

In Brazil, I witnessed such an event and the woman next to me received her Orixá. After several hours of watching drumming and dancing, the woman fell into a swoon. I tried to help her, but two people from the temple efficiently came over and lifted her out of her chair and took her into the back room, where she was fitted with the Orixá's costume, and tested through different rhythms and dances that she spontaneously moved to and that showed her teachers which Orixá was emerging. The rest of us "tourists" were dismissed immediately. At this point it was well after midnight, and I imagined she would be in process for sometime after we all left. These ceremonies often go on all night and into the next day. Most of the initiations I witnessed went on for several days.

In *Heart Path*, I have a section on page 55 where I go into greater detail about the sixteen Umbanda Orixás and what they mean. If one wants to learn more about Orixás, I suggest you start there first. Then there are many other books that may attract you on the topic. Ultimately going into your own heart and learning what elements are present is one way to discover your essence. Here is another way to discover more of your self:

For your clients, sometimes behaviors they have are an outgrowth of the Orixá and not necessary pathological. An example of this is my friend the Ogum, a river of movement who could be mistaken for a "type A" personality.

Ether the 8th Element – There exists in the universe a substance that lives between and through all things. It is known in Native American circles as The Great Mother, or Star Woman, it is known by scientist as aluminiferous ether[14] or etheric matter[15]. In Eastern religion it is called "subtle matter"[16]. Those interested in Spirituality and the Occult sciences know it as ether. In the Oxford American Dictionary the term *ether* began to appear in the 17th century, referring to the substance or life force that lives between air, which cannot be felt or seen, but can be experienced. However, the term goes back to Aristotle who invented the word, which he used for substance of the universe.[17] In the Miriam Webster Dictionary, the definition is: "1: a medium that in the wave theory of light permeates all space and transmits transverse waves."[18]

14   Hawkins, Stephen and Leonard Mlodinow, *The Grand Design*, Bantam Books, New York, pgs.94-96.
15   Gerber, Richard, *Vibrational Medicine*, Bear & Co, Rochester, Vt. pg. 60, 156
16   ibid, pg. 60
17   Hawkins, Stephen, Leonard Mlodinow, *The Grand Design*, Bantam Books, New York, pg. 93
18   Miriam Webster Dictionary, on-line www.miriamwebster.com

It is the awareness of this substance in the Universe that helps psychics connect to what is often called the universal grid-work as illustrated by Alex Grey in his phenomenal book, *Sacred Mirrors*.[19] This grid-work connects all things to all things. It is the matter that is of a higher vibration than physical matter. It also is why one can perceive things long distance. It is how I or any psychic can perceive and 'read' aura's long distance. This same etheric matter is used to help people heal when the right intention and vibration is sent to it.

As I said before, in Energy Medicine, a practitioner works with energy. In Energy Medicine, you use your intention and the intention of the client to rebalance and reverse disease.

Sometimes when I assist in someone's healing, I actually create things out of the ether and help people with various constructions that I place in their field to help them shift long held patterns. When you do guided imagery, you work with this energy whether you know it or not. Emotions, thoughts and intentions are transmitted by ethereal energy. Guided imagery also works on a deep soul level. The spontaneous images a person receives are an indication that they are connecting on a deeper level than thought. They are engaging the soul and effecting deep internal change.

In one example a 64-year-old man came in with a chronic tightness in his right hip. He was a client I have worked with many times with other problems that we had cleared up over time as a result of our work together. This time he had tightness in his hip that he reported for the first time to me he had had for over 10 years. In the process of working with this pain he had visited Chiropractors, Physicians, Orthopedic doctors, and nothing seemed to relieve the tightness. He practiced Chi-gung and Tai Chi, and he found this block severely inhibited his movement. When he brought this challenge to me, we were able to clear it up in one session.

After gathering his inner family together, I had him bring the energy to the outside of the heart garden. He perceived a block, like stone, that was being held there. My image was of a man bent over and bearing down with teeth bared like an Aztec or Mayan sculpture of a male figure giving birth. Since he was an artist, he was familiar with the sculpture I was describing, and he was able to pinpoint the problem; he was trying too hard to give birth to himself.

19   Grey, Alex. *Sacred Mirrors*, Inner Traditions International, NY, 1990.

I then asked that he send this image love, and he dissolved the image of the stone. I asked if I could further help his healing by doing some Energy Medicine in the joint. This work extends beyond the Heart Path process, and is used to help him release the pattern entirely. As he agreed for me to do more work on him, out of the ether, I placed what I call an 'isotope,' which if I could manifest it, looks like a clear fiber-optic rod that brings light into the joint. I placed this into his hip chakra (a minor chakra from the side of the hip going into the second chakra from each side) with the intent of keeping this channel open. I set in the rod an intention to last 2 weeks, as that would get him through enough of his daily cycles not to contract into the pattern again. When he left the session, he could feel that he was much freer in his hip. Before he left my office, he did a move from Tai Chi, and his eyes widened, and he laughed out loud! "Wow, he said, I have not been able to move like this for years!" I told him what I did, and that it should give him enough time to correct the problem. His job in the next few weeks was to notice how he contracted that hip and to stay aware of the pattern that would want to contract back into the old 'trying too hard' mode of being.

I find that using ether consciously gives me a way to support the person quietly, subtly, and without pain or side effects. When I do use it, I always tell them about it, so if their system is not comfortable with the 'isotope' then they can remove it themselves, though this has never happened as far as I know. Like my client, they are usually so glad to have relief, they are more than happy to have me do whatever will help them.

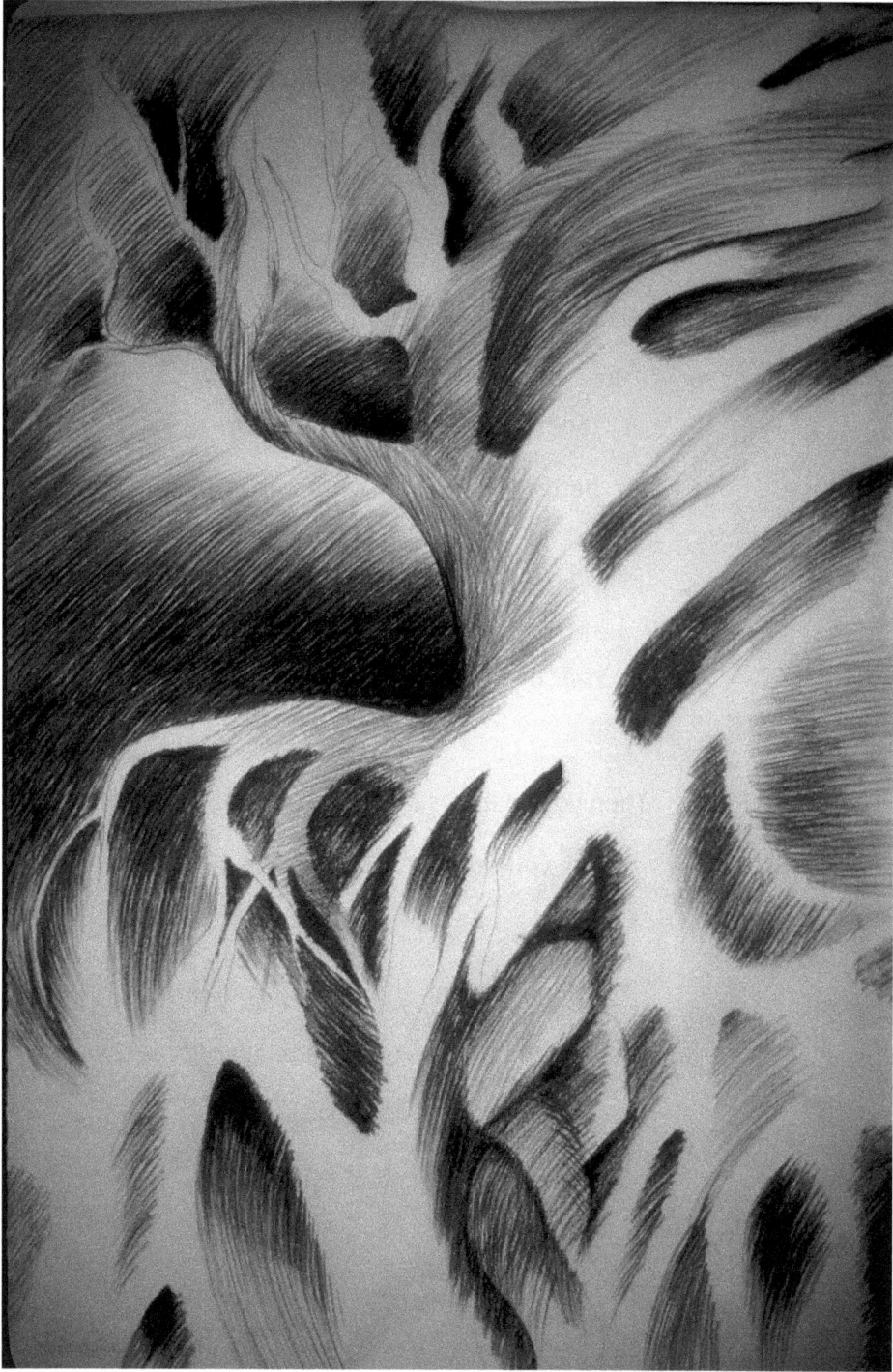

Light Roots / Family Tree - Charcoal Painting
by the Author

Chapter 3 – Keys to Healing the self into Self
Ways to Use Heart Path

<u>Vista</u>

Friend, whose eyes

are you looking through?

See with your mountain eyes,

better yet the lion, or the dove.

Embrace the crying child

stand on your head if you have to get his attention,

Then your parents in there can hold her

while you notice two essert flowers

Breaking through the crust of rubble

and the face that loves you despite everything

shining brighter than the Sun.

A Word about Wounding and Separation

Now that you have the basic mediation, and know the elements of what these archetypes and the

Three Stars mean, let's continue to look at what wounding actually is, and how it can be healed. Of course

we know that wounding has to be seen before it can be healed. But taking a moment to view wounding in

another light can be very helpful when thinking about what issues the client presents.

Many Hindu and Buddhist[20] teachers will tell you that all pain stems from separation from Source. This separation is an individual as well as collective wound. If you think about ways people are wounded, namely through betrayal, abandonment or rejection, all three have their roots in separation. Separation is often expressed in fear *or* anger, or fear *and* anger, both of which have their roots in the belief of separation.

Stepping back from this statement from Buddhist and Hindu teachers, I would say that dis-ease occurs for many reasons that we do not fully comprehend. For example we know that chemicals in the environment create cancers and other illnesses. Disease can occur from karma and from other illnesses.

As an example, if someone is separated from either parent at a young age, there often will be wounds of abandonment by the parent that left. Parents are seen as source, as Gods, for the child. They are gods that provide everything for them until they can provide it for themselves. However, the child takes that in as a personal affront and believes it is their fault, often with a belief about them selves namely; "I'm not good enough" or "It's my fault they left, or I am not loveable." These beliefs cause more pain, they cause more separation. It feeds the collective wound. However, if abandonment is the issue, for example, the person has, in some way, already abandoned themselves. The person outside them has only recreated what was already taken place inside.

An example of this was a woman client, 58 year old, who had not had children and unconsciously beat herself up for not having them. She did not know that wound was there until she commented on how one of her friend's children was misbehaving once again in a group setting. The client's friend and her child had discussed this with a larger group many times, and still the behavior was not corrected. The 'friend' grew angry and slashed her back with the retort 'you don't even *have* children.' That retort was not what harmed the client, it was her own self-wounding around motherhood that was really hurting her. When she came to see me, she was hurting badly. What I 'saw' was the wound of her own self-hatred 'eating

---

20   Thick Nat Han, *Learning How to Love*, CD's

her up.' (It looked like glass teeth that were attaching her heart chakra.) Once these 'teeth'
were brought to consciousness, the healing could take place. This occurred in one session
after the incident with her 'friend.'

Addressing separation, gives the client perspective, the recognition of where the
wound is stemming from, and then what belief systems underlay the wound. This client
mentioned in the previous paragraph, had the belief that she had failed. "I don't have children
so therefore I am not enough." When she released this belief, she found a way to forgive the
person and herself. Often a huge release and feeling of freedom follows. Sometimes these old
beliefs resurface at various times in a person's life. The wounded one works unconsciously to
reinforce the original "I'm not good enough" belief system on different levels. The person may
sometimes attract similar wounding situations in order to release the wound. This attraction
pushes the right combination of wounding "buttons" to activate the wound so it can be felt.
With the Heart Path meditation once the inner family is present within your client, you can
ask if there are any aspects that are outside of the heart garden that need to come in. This is
a way to find the abandon parts that may be working unconsciously against the person and
need to be brought inside the heart garden where 'all work together as one'. Once inside the
garden, there are ways to release old behaviors, beliefs, and anger or fear that prevent them
connecting more fully with life around them. Helping the client see that this belief is; a) not
true, b) no longer useful; and c) creates pain for them, the client is then ready to release the
belief, pain or pattern to reintegrate the energy. Because a pattern of behavior or thought
takes energy to construct and maintain, there is always a release of energy when healing
takes place. Sometimes a person feels lighter, and sometimes they feel tired if it has been
emotionally challenging for them.

Releasing the Old Patterns

One of the most effective ways to release these old patterns is to have the client
imagine that inside the heart garden is a campfire that his or her inner family gathers around.
This was mentioned previously on page 14. When the aspect that was wounded is ready, the

client can release all these old patterns into the fire. One way to do it is if they imagine them a spider web or an old map that gets released into the fire. The aspect that created it can extract the pattern and let it go. However the aspect of self 'sees' the pattern and release of it, is up to them and often presents itself in fascinating ways, including suits of clothes, armor, etc.

It is amazing to me the variety of visual ways that the person can let go of 'patterns.' One client saw the pattern as spaghetti cords that she was taking out of the body. Others see them as wiring or cording, yet another might see it as roads or as a map plan, or contract to be released.

They may have another way to release the pattern, but the fire is a primal beginning element of destruction and renewal and it regenerates the energy of the person to let go of the pattern. Once the pattern is destroyed and the energy released, the person will feel lighter, freer and happier with more energy available to them. Remember that energy cannot be created or destroyed, it just is. In Energy Medicine the practitioner often assists in the energy transforming from one place to another.

They also may have a moment of fear before they release it. This is natural if the pattern has acted as a boundary for others. However, you can ask if there is a way they can have boundaries without congesting their systems with all this wiring. Usually they will come up with another way. Often times, if they are at a loss, you can ask them to simply say 'no' to the person with whom they need to create a boundary.

Old patterns are just like a diversionary circuit board, where energy is siphoned off from a main circuit board in order to 'run' a separate program, and it takes life force energy away from the essence of living. You can think of it like downloading more programs into your computer, which takes up space on your hard drive. It is what the ego does, creates more patterns to use up the energy of the person to redirect life force to feed itself. Once these old useless patterns are released the energy of the person is freed up to use in other ways.

The process is working when there is a release of energy and the client feels more liberated as a result. Once they have released their own patterns, one might address issues of forgiveness that can assist in healing the relationship with the parent or person with whom they are in conflict.

Whether the client is in contact with the person or not, alive or dead, the forgiveness by the client will liberate the client. This helps everybody and loosens the knot of the collective separation. Truly, when we heal ourselves we heal the world.

Forgiveness as a Key to Liberation

Forgiveness is so important. It releases karmic knots of wounding, and helps everyone move into more freedom as the client progresses in their process. But how do you guide the client to forgive what appear often to be serious wounds? Even if the person knows the wound is theirs, and they have been working on it, often forgiveness is not easy.

The answer is to check in with them about it. Forgiveness has to be done on their timing even if they know they need to do it. Sometimes they just can't (or won't) until they have gotten to the point where they see that holding on to anger or sadness just keeps them separate from themselves, and creates punishment of the self and the other person. They can only release the old if they feel it to be right for them. When they get to that point you can be ready with the following questions:

More Key Questions on Forgiveness:

a) Are you ready to release all of this old wounding?

b) Can you forgive your (father, mother, offending party)?

c) Can you forgive yourself for being related to them? (Or contracting with that person for this lesson?)

d) If not what are you getting out of holding on to the anger, wound or incident?

Here is something that one of my guides whispered to me recently after experiencing a blast from a person that was close to me. The result was that I surrendered more deeply into my own wounding and released some basic beliefs that were hurting all my relationships.

"No one can hurt you." The Ancient Ones said.

Whee!!! This was a revelation. Wait a minute!!! Had I not just stood there while an angry wind rushed over me from an offended party?

"Yes, but they did not hurt you, this is an old wound that they activated, just as you activated their wound, which is why they were angry in the first place. You were wounding yourself and the pain was made visible by you wounding them."

When I sat still in mediation, I had found the self-hating part that was angry at me for not being what I had always dreamed myself to be. As I asked for help, the section of myself that was wounding me, let go through the help of my spiritual guidance. These 'Grandmothers' were amazingly helpful.

Clients that have wounds "inflicted on them" often have some kind of past life connection where they injured the offending party in a past incarnation. If we go deep enough into the patterns one can see them as interlocking spirals strands of light through time. Just like our DNA, these strands form a double helix of balance. Sometimes, if the wounds are severe enough, a person will dissolve that 'partnership of relating.' Then they will find more harmonious and less damaging relationships. This can be set through their internal agreements with their inner family usually at the end of a session. I do this as it arises in the questioning and not as a matter of course in every session. I ask the client to imagine their agreement with the person to be 'un-scrolled' before them so they can see what they agreed to. Often the agreements are gone, completed, or no longer in operation. Clients can then agree or disagree with more contact. Often they agree to continue loving them without attachments. Once the agreements are re-evaluated the client can start fresh with that person or release the relationship.

When people are evolving, often there are breaks with their old relational group. You see this often with people who are leaving addiction and forming healthier relationships through Alcoholics Anonymous and other such groups. These double helixes will break apart and they will find others to connect with to carry on their life lessons. Setting intentions for better relating is very helpful. Remembering love, trust, respect and good communication is essential to reform commitments.

Attachments and Love

Love and attachment often get confused in relationships. Love and attachment are very important especially in early childhood development when attachment for children to mothers and fathers are necessary for their security and sense of place within the family. However, as children grow up, those attachments become unhealthy if they are still there beyond the needs of the child. Parents often remain attached as they have given their lives to their children, and once they have done this, it is hard to shift their perspectives, especially if they have invested a great deal of identity into parenting. Children too, often take longer to grow up, and it is a wise parent who moves them along rather than holds on to them. Energetically cording develops between people. When there is a cord attached, it feels as though someone has you on a string. This is literally true. Those 'strings' are the cords, and they are mostly quite unhealthy. Real love gives one a sense of freedom to be all they can be. It gives freely and doesn't expect payback—or in some cases—a pound of flesh.

When clients come in who are parents, I always ask the age of their children. Sometimes the way they speak is as if the children are quite small. But when I discover they are over 30, then it is time to talk to the parent about letting go of the attachment to their children. The love will always be there, but the attachment does not have to be.

Releasing cording does not negate agreements of children to take care of parents in their older age. Nor does it have to cancel commitment to always be there for each other when things get tough in life. However, the feelings of obligation mixed with cords and love are sometimes very toxic indeed.

When a client is ready to release attachments, and be love, the cords can be released and the love remains. In the next chapter I will speak more about cording and how to release them.

Current time

As mentioned previously past lives do crop up if the therapist is willing or able to deal with them in a session. However, all issues of the past whether ten years ago or a hundred are present in the moment. Diving into the moment and staying current with emotions as they arise, especially core issues, beliefs, etc., can heal past lives as well. Past lives emerge in current time healing and often have really old unconscious beliefs attached to them.

Sometimes these lives emerge as figures from the past dressed in period dress standing around outside the heart garden. Often when I see a past life, I ask the aspect why they are there. Direct questions work best such as; *who are you?*; *Are you from a past life?*; or *Are you a separate entity?* Sometimes an entity attaches to the client at the point of grief such as the root chakra, the second chakra, or solar-plexus chakra. In this case, ask the entity to leave the client. Usually not much else is required. Sometimes, if you ask an angel or Mother Mary or Kwan Yin to come in and take the entity, that helps the client release responsibility for them. Most often the client is already presenting and speaking about past lives when they come in for a session. A sure sign of a past life issue emerging for healing is if the client is feeling overwhelmed – in an out of proportioned way – to what is currently emotionally taxing. If the client does not believe in past lives, there is no sense in going into it. The best course then is to work currently with their emotional issues in present time and declare this healing for all time and space.

Spiritual Health: What is it to be spiritually healthy?

Basically we are all in a process of moving towards more spiritual health. I would define being spiritually healthy as living in the core of your being, living from the knowledge and experience of being loved and connected to the Earth and the Heavens. It is living with humility and confidence that you belong here, and that you are love.

This spiritual health has to do with your vertical alignment in the body. In the physical body, in front of the spine, you have the core of your being running through and encompassing the entire energy system. As you grow in spiritual centeredness, you grow in love, compassion and well being. This core, which may be felt as a stream of light or life force running though the body, expands as you develop your spiritual wisdom and light. It helps on every level of being to maintain optimal health and wellness. This light is your essence, and it is the love that opens to the "Great Love" that Rumi suggested in the poem in the first chapter.

Maintaining a Spiritual Practice to Maintain Spiritual Health

When you meditate, pray, or take time to rebalance the self through exercises such as walking or biking, you bring yourself into alignment with your core. Meditation is the oldest and most reliable form of being present with the self. It has a history that goes back to the Buddha and beyond. In addition it works! The more you consistently meditate daily, and length of time does not seem as important as consistence, the more you gain a chain of wellness in your connection to all that is. Every time you meditate you connect the links in this chain. What happens in my experience is that you begin to realize that you have a core and centered self. Heart Path helps people come into that center and begin to feel it. The Heart Garden helps raise awareness from power struggles to the heart and connection with All-That-Is.

Maintaining a spiritual practice helps your whole being. It revitalizes your sense of centeredness, and helps your whole system maintain energy. Combined with exercise as in a walking meditation, it helps each person feel and maintain spiritual health.

Causes of Spiritual Illness, Soul-loss

When a person is not aware of centering, not interested in their connection to nature or the world around them, they are not very spiritually healthy. If they use drugs and substances to self-medicate, they are not very healthy on any level. The loss of faith and loss of belief in something greater than one's self are all contributors to an unhealthy spiritual self.

When a person isolates from lack of being able or willing to engage the world, sometimes, unless they are engaging the world through the solitude necessary to create art, music or other forms of connecting deep within the self, the person can become energetically clogged up and on many levels and will exhibit ill health. It goes without saying that spiritual ill-health can be caused by drugs, alcohol, or other substance abuse.

Soul loss occurs when a wound occurs, such as abandonment, physical attach, or emotional attach, or other injury. When a child is hurt, say by abuse either physical or emotional, a part of them breaks off and keeps trying to figure out what happened to cause this to happen. Especially if the person is hurt through death or things outside of their control, there is soul-loss when the part stays at that age to try and work it out. This divides the flow of energy. As the soul aspects are returned, as through shamanic practices and or through using the Heart Path process, the person feels more energy returning through the integration of this aspect of the self. Forgiveness and clearer understanding helps to bring this about. Also calling forth the person's aspect that was left, the 4 year old or 7 year old, to the heart garden gate, the person can witness and bring home the part that was left behind. In my work with people, I use this process to help return the energy back to the self of the client.

Other problems that people face with soul-loss has to do with making deals with other entities that are not here for the best and highest good of the client. People open "portals" in the self unknowingly. In once case, a 42-year-old client came to see me with entities attaching her. When she was a teenager, she played around with a Ouija Board with friends at a slumber party. Unknowingly she opened a portal in her own energy field and ever since had problems with entities. What she did was open a doorway to the self that she was not able to control or manage. In our single session, I closed the "Portals" after sending those entities back to where they came from and sealed the doors in her root chakra. I also cleared off other energies that were attached to her fear, and got her into her center and grounded so that they did not bother her. I also explained that if she was fully occupying herself, nothing else could or would. When she left my office, she was balanced, grounded and entity free.

Some entities and people are so identified with their lack of love or their negative aspects that they think they are worthless or worse 'not of the light'. When this is the case, and someone has entities that attach them, they often are afraid to an extreme, and often their own lack of identity with the love that they are, is lacking almost entirely. The entities "match" the fear of that which attacks them. I work to bring the client's well being into alignment through first aligning with the light, as in the three stars meditation, then releasing negative beliefs into the bon fire within the heart garden process. I clear off the entities, sending them to the Earth or the light, and demand without fear that they leave. If they refuse or try to come back, I call in the Counsel of High Beings and Archangels, and have them deal with the entity. Then I talk to the client about releasing their fear of these entities by having them realize that these entities are really here to help them let go of their fear. My experience is that negative entities are actually here in the service of health and wholeness by reflecting to us where our fears lie. When we can clear them, the entities have nothing to hold on to and the "attacks" stop.

In extreme cases, some clients like the drama of these attacks. Sometimes they are manifestations of their own mind, sometimes there are real entities that attack them. Sometimes these "entities" are parts of their own psyche that are attacking them out of self-hatred. To discern all this is sometimes challenging, but it can be done, and often when the process of healing is complete, that is when a client feels the shift after a session.

This topic could be a whole book on energetic releases with the astral plane, and other such negative places in the self, but this is as much as I want to cover in this book at this time.

Mental Health: From any perspective, mental health is maintained by self-love and connection to All That Is. When a person has healthy relationships and has healthy self-love, there is nothing wrong with them. When a person divides the self to cope with trauma, such as in schizophrenia or has chemical imbalances such as in a bi-polar condition, the mental health of the person is considered pathological in Western Psychology.

My perception about schizophrenia is that the psyche has taken care of itself by dividing up the soul or energy of the person so as not to have it killed or destroyed. A person can be healed in some cases, with a skilled therapist. While this can be done over time, most people who are diagnosed with this condition are not financially able to have a therapist help them. Many of the cases of people I have encountered are people who are extremely poor, in jail, on the street with no financial means of support. Our mental health system is a shambles and does little to help them heal.

In some cases, I have used Heart Path to help a person who was so deeply abused that they split into fragments of self. I discuss this in future pages of the book.

Wounding and separation cause mental illness as stated in the beginning of this chapter. If we can recognize our wounds and places in us that are separate, we can heal them. Various mental patterns and belief systems create suffering and faulty beliefs about the self. Changing these are not as hard as one might think. A person just has to become conscious of the wounding and begin to heal by correcting the beliefs. A person might do this by being vigilant about the belief, and keep noticing when it comes up. Then with the aspect of the self identified who holds that belief, the person might bring the aspect to the heart garden or notice it's activity inside, and let go of the belief that keeps them separate. The problem with a belief that is not healthy such as the one previously discussed of the 58 year old woman who had the belief that she was not worthy because she did not have children, that when someone has such a belief, it attracts others who are going to activate it. In our culture, that is so family orientated and the "norm" is to have children, it can be hard to not be wounded repeatedly by other's families. But if the wound is handled at a deep level, then, as in the case with this woman, she was able to release the wounding and now feels fine about not having children. Actually as an artist and writer, she is happy not to have them so she can explore her work freely in these areas.

Identifying Faulty Belief Systems

Some beliefs that are common are: I am not good enough, I am not worthy of love, I am a bad person, I have to do it alone, I can't receive love, and many others. The primary ones that hold people hostage, especially women, is I am not good enough. Also patterns of martyrdom, or Victim/Perpetrator are also ways that people create negative patterns of relating and negative dynamics in all aspects of their lives. In the next chapter I will deal with ego-based patterns that keep us from feeling love and unity. The topic really needs its own chapter.

Anxiety – For some anxiety is caused by the belief that a person is not safe. This is definitely a fear-based pattern. Safety is created by self-love. So when working with a person in a session, the anxiety can be released through the bon fire. It really works. Also the pattern of anxiety in the nervous system is the "default mechanism" for releasing nervous energy. I use the fire to dump the excess energy, and then call the "nervous Nelly or Ned" to the Heart Garden gate. When the client witnesses the one causing the anxiety, and then witnesses that there are other parts that are not nervous, this helps a lot to release anxiety. Sometimes what is needed is to ask what the nervous aspect is worried about. When they explain the fundamental nervousness, or lack of trust of the self, then sometimes the inner-self can make compromises. It always helps to bring the nervous one inside to the heart garden. Sometimes I discuss with the client the nerve wracking situations in their lives and help them release those situations through a) acknowledging the situation, b) problem solving ways to be in relationship with others that create the nervousness. c) releasing the victim perpetrator dynamic (see Chapter 4).

In one case, a 34-year-old woman came to see me. She was full of anxiety and did not know why. When we discussed her work life she revealed that she was being changed from one department to another. This had not happened in her work-life and it was very anxiety producing. When we examined the situation of her work-life, we decided that her position was assured. This was done both by questioning her and by looking at the flow of energy through psychic perception. When we did the Heart Garden process, we discovered a 10 year old, 19 year old, a 20 year old and a 24 year old that were all really anxious about transitions that she had previously gone through at those ages. The 10 year old was the first one, during her parents' divorce, who began feeling anxious. Then the 19 year old who was deciding what to do with her life, was also terrified of getting out into the world. Then the 20 year old was beginning her working life and had a relationship break-up. The 24 year old got divorced.

At each transition her nervous system was activated to experience anxiety, and because not one of the previous ages of anxiety had been resolved, they added more anxiety on top of the previous experience. In a one-hour session, we were able to bring these aspects to the outside of the heart garden, lining them up outside when I asked the questions "who is creating anxiety for you." Beginning with the youngest aspect, she told me her story, and I acknowledged the trauma she must have felt. Then I asked if she knew she was not age 10 but now had an inner family that would never and could never leave. As we worked through the reality of each of the aspects being in the past, we brought the energy of the various ages into the heart garden. At each stage we reinforced the fact that the anxiety was not helpful, and that the belief in lack of safety was released. We grew up the 10 year old through her teens to her late teens through the 19 year old to the 20 year old to the 24 year old and finally made it to the 34-year-old present time adult.

As a side note to this case, this woman had received therapy around her parents divorce for a number of years in her mid-twenties. As a result she had already laid the groundwork for the work we did together. However, I have done this exact process with others with anxiety, releasing the nervousness into the heart garden bon fire and it works every time. It also gives the client a way to manage their own nervous systems when they can't get help. Also the belief in lack of safety is released so that there is no need to keep feeling unsafe. Lack of safety is a state of mind, often caused by an experience that the ego then must keep attracting or keep perceiving, even if the person is perfectly safe in reality. This way the ego proves to the person, that the lack of safety is real and justified. This is what the ego does to "prove it is right." "Proving one to be right" is in itself another ego pattern.

Depression-When I perceive someone's system that is depressed, often what I 'see' is oppression or suppression. Sometimes in the field, there is a literal plunger in the field that pushes down a person's aura in the 1st, 2nd, or 3rd chakra or in all three. This suppression is sometimes related to familial lines, such as in people that have been repressed, such as in Native Americans or people of color, however it can also occur in women, and in people who have experienced oppression within their family groups. In two cases, I have seen this pattern in Native American women. One client, who I saw in jail, had an entire family in her generation of drug-addicted siblings. All 10 of them were addicted to heroine, crack, or cocaine. Ironically her aging parents did not drink or smoke or use anything. When questioning her further, she said her grandfather had been captured and taken off his land in Southern California and enslaved by one of the Missions. He became alcoholic, and his son (her father) vowed not to drink. However, the reason the grandfather became alcoholic was the powerlessness over the removal and enslavement he experienced. All that grief and feeling of failure, going from a free person to a captured one, had never been allowed to be processed. Furthermore her mother, being a good catholic, followed in the practices of the oppressor. Her race was part Native American and part Mexican American. So, the kids were all expressing their grief and sadness over this issue, not to mention confusion.

Another 43-year-old woman who was of mixed race ancestry, came in with thoughts of suicide, and was quite depressed. I took her on to see if we could shift the depression. She was also under the care of a therapist. As I looked at her field, she had this plunger in her system that pushed her energy down. (I have seen this in many people with depression). After she described her feelings, when I brought the plunger to her attention, my perception only confirmed her experience. Over time we began to release the pattern, which in this case was a huge plunger of "not good enough".

Her European (mostly German) American mother was quite narcissistic and her father was the Native American lineage that felt oppressed in his relationship with her. She and a brother were often left to fend for themselves, and there was a divorce early on in her childhood. The grief of her ancestry and guilt of the European ancestry, was expressing itself through her. As she became more involved in the traditions of her Native American ancestry, she felt better about herself. We worked together in hour-long sessions every other week for a period of one year. When we started working together, she had decided to go off her depression meds for a year to see how she faired. This was done independently of my treatment with her and her work with a therapist, with whom she was also working. At the end of a year, she felt better, though during times of challenge she was still not relieved of all her depression symptoms. Her chemical imbalance was still there. She decided to take the meds again during the time of one transition, job change, moving, kids moving out, which all happened at one time. Afterwards she tapered off and got more engaged in crafts, which helped her self-esteem and she began to feel better about herself. Her kids started having grandkids, and this engaged her as well. She felt more needed and useful in her life. Her father had passed away, and her mother remarried. She decided it was not helpful for her to be in contact with her mother, so she cut ties. At last report she was taking only a very small dose of her medication and able to maintain her emotional health with less depression and more joy.

Emotional Healing-How to Handle Emotions as Indicators

Our emotions are the place where our spirit and our bodies meet. You could say "where the rubber of our experiences meets the road of our bodies." The emotions are our barometer of what is going on in the self. Anger is the most common, and often it is an indication of boundaries crossed or unresolved anger at the past. When someone is angry about something, it means "Get out! You have no business here!!" Anger can also indicate betrayal or neglect. Throwing the anger in the internal fire is one way to handle releasing it as previously mentioned. Another way is to speak to the offending party 'over the fence.' The garden gate is useful in drawing a boundary. When someone has crossed that boundary, I often ask the person to call that person forward and ask that they speak about their boundary and how they feel about it to the person. They speak, and then they listen to the other person, keeping them outside their heart garden. If the person is perceived as dangerous or mean, I call in the allies of the client to surround them and also the animal nature to stand on either side of speaker in the heart garden. This gives the client support.

When the conversation is over, the client often reports to me what has gone on inside them, and there is usually some sort of resolution, new boundaries drawn and the forgiveness work has been completed. The person is released from the old pattern of the past. I always review what the client came in for in the first place, and often refer back to what was needed by the client and their relationship to the past life to close the session. This gives them a clear understanding of where they have been and where they are going. I validate them for their progress and remind them if necessary that they can say anything as long as it comes from the heart. However violence or further fighting is not good to continue internally or externally. If they get into a fight with the person inside themselves, I would suggest becoming a full-fledged referee. Bringing in the image of a referee can lighten the tension, and call a 'fair' game. It is surprising to me how well this works. It also lightens up the atmosphere.

In one case, a 37-year-old man called me to clear out his house. "I have an entity in here, and it wakes me up every night. I can't sleep." When I went over to his home, there was a great deal of chaos in his house. I talked with him about chaos and entities, that they often enter houses where there is a lot of it. After clearing out the energy, I had a feeling that the entity was going to come back. This almost never happens. However, I told him if it come back to call me right away. A week later it did return. In the second session I could perceive that this "entity" was a part of him that was really angry at him. Over the course of that session we integrated that angry part. However, that was just the beginning. The man had had a spiritual opening of great proportions prior to my first visit. He felt the great emptiness, the great fullness and wanted to change and surrender to the light. Over the course of a year working every month, 12 sessions, we cleared up many past lives that were not so wonderful. He had to confront himself as a gangster, a murderer, a slave, a dictator, and over time he integrated these lives, released their need to control everyone and everything. He has transformed his identity as a scoundrel into that of a loving and compassionate man that he knows as his true nature. He also moved out of his house and followed his bliss to Colorado where he lives today.

In the case of Doris, the 44 year old with the desire to have a mate who had misinterpreted beliefs from her mother, she saw her fear of relationship and her beliefs as spaghetti wiring that was impacting her system. We dissolved them by putting them into the fire. She spent the last part of her last session pulling out the old 'wiring.'

In the film, "What the Bleep Do We Know" Candice Pert, author of the landmark book *Molecules of Emotion* describes exactly what happened here. As our emotions get a signal of fear or anger, we trigger the old beliefs that release peptides into the system that unlock the chemical pattern we become used to, namely fear or anger. As we shift our beliefs so to we shift those neuro-pathways and the peptides get another signal. My client ingeniously saw these pathways as spaghetti coming out of her system when she released the old beliefs into the fire, "I am better off alone" and agreed internally with all her aspects that "I am worthy of love and I deserve a loving relationship with a man."

Facing Fears and Dissolving Them

Heart Path works wonders with fear of all kinds. Many people are facing huge fears of interacting, relating, being out in the world, or just plain surviving on Mother Earth. They are afraid of life and living it. Usually they are afraid as a survival strategy. One of my teachers Da Free John, said once (paraphrasing as I heard it in a lecture) there are three kinds of persons, a vital (anger-based person) a solid (fear-based person) or peculiar (fear and anger-based combination). I was offended when I first heard this, of course my ego didn't like it much, but I realized over time, that it was a very profound teaching of how our egos strategize to cover the base of existence. Over time I have learned that our task is to release our survival strategies to convert that fear and/or anger base into love. Then we are not the victim nor the perpetrator, but the loving witness of life force flowing through us. We become empty of strategy and live our lives freely in the flow of life living us.

Perceiving a client's fears is often exhibited in overt body language. Energetically fear 'looks' like cement, often white in color, cement in texture, or it can be perceived as calcification or as in the case of Doris, white spaghetti wires. (If not dealt with in the body, it becomes arthritis, or stiffness in tissues or joints or other diseases.) However, you do not have to be psychic to perceive fear in someone. We know it when we see it in their posture and way of being. Sometimes people come in a straight jacket of fear, and walk or move very stiffly.

Usually, recognizing the purpose of the fear, that is protection of the self, is helpful when releasing it. However, the truth about fear is that only attracts what the person *does not* want. This occurs as part of the natural fight or flight mechanism of the body. It is an exaggerated extension of the animal nature. Often I see that, no matter how mean the inner critics or angry and venting a part can be, their underlying motivation is usually one of loving us and working towards wholeness. Some inner critics use criticism to get the best out of us. However, it rarely works well because the best we can be is done lovingly not fearfully. Their methods, once pointed out, give the critic perspective to change behaviors that do not work. There is something that person is trying to tell them or something they are trying to learn. Once the client realizes that fear is not helpful and it only draws to one what one is afraid of, they realize it does help to let it go. Fear does not help us evolve beyond it. The fear of the unknown is usually the biggest one we have to overcome. In the Heart Path process, it is helpful to let go of fears into the fire or send love to the fear. The person also must realize new ways to cope with fear as it arises, such as putting fears into the fire, or calling in an animal aspect that isn't afraid of anything. Freedom from fear is a great gift. The world is a loving place if we choose it to be, especially if we can release our fear and live in love.

Healing Anger

As mentioned previously, anger is another survival strategy. It helps to recognize it for what it is. It is also an indication of crossed boundaries in personal relationships. When there are no boundaries with others, one can feel violated. As a survival strategy it often fuels a person into and out of experiences. It can also be a way to get people away from them in intimate relationships. As a reaction, it is part of the victim/perpetrator dynamic. Anger is the result. When a client with a clear channel of anger vents it in a session, what I often do is acknowledge it first "I hear you are really angry." Then we find the violation in the relationships. Again, the bon fire works wonders to release the rage. Often there is a string of violations prior to this anger arising. As in the previous woman with several ages of unresolved anxiety, you can move through the anger ages, and release the root causes. You can also find the underlying belief to the strategy of anger as a survival strategy. In some cases, especially in men, the client probably inherited this strategy from the father. Sometimes it can be the mother, but rarely, it is usually the father that was angry and passed down the behavior to his son. Once the client is conscious of it as a pattern, they can work with it and release it.

In one case, a 72-year-old man who had a history of resorting to anger, came to see me. He recognized that his 8 year old was the one who really began this pattern, learning it from his father. When we were able to be with his inner 8 year old, the child was in a full tantrum. At that time he was 8, his father had been abusive and angry after a night drinking. He hit the child and abused the mother. The son witnessed this. It made him extremely angry. But because the child had no recourse, he held onto the anger, and only later was able to express it as he got big enough to defend himself. He decided then and there that he had to take care of himself because no one else, not mother nor father, would or could. Ever since the 8 year old was taking control! He controlled others with his anger.

As we worked with the child together, his adult self said: "This kid is a real brat." When I pointed out to him that self-judgment doesn't help anything, he realized how he had become the "abusing" father to his own inner child. Name-calling is one of the things his own father did frequently. He was able to realize this on his own, and soon he was able to reconcile with his inner child. He released a ton of anger in that session, and left with enough tools to help himself shift. I also had him "arrest" his 8 year old from responsibility of being "the one who had to do it all." We let go of that belief, as the child recognized that his inner parents were there for him. He cried throughout the session as these had been knots in his psyche that kept him from moving forward in his life.

Grief

One of the most powerful all-encompassing experience one can have is grief. All of the emotions cycle, anger, denial, fear, resentment, depression, acceptance, and then it starts all over again. Grief is also one of those experiences that puts you in another world from others, and can create a huge amount of separation in the self from the world.

Much of the work I do as a medium is to help people process their grief and resolve past experiences with loved ones who have died. Having gone through many death experiences myself with those who I loved and still love very much, has actually helped me sit with others in their pain. However, everyone processes grief differently, and some may take years to resolve a loss while others move towards acceptance rather quickly.

Sometimes grief gets piled on top of grief. When someone has multiple deaths in a short time frame, it can cause more trauma. Greater attachment to those who are left can occur. Also greater fears and paranoia can also set in.

The thing that helped me the most was going through grief groups with the Hospice Bereavement program. I often suggest it for clients. I also remind them that grief takes the time it takes. There is no rushing the process. However, I know what helped me the most was the determination to feel my feelings. Whenever the grief arose I allowed as best I could to feel it.

Often I hated the feelings, and also had to learn more compassion for myself. But I did not shirk my responsibility to feel through the pain until it did not hurt so much. I did this with the deaths of my mother, daughter, sister, and marriage. Loss can occur in many ways and needs to be processed by most people. That is why I often recommend personal rituals for transition for times of moving, career change, loss of homes, divorce, moving, etc. My first book, Dancing Up the Moon, (Conari Press) is soon to be published in a new volume called Ceremonies from the Heart, For Children, Adults and the Earth (Blue Bone Books). This book suggests rituals for all occasions.

Physical Health and Illness

Everyone knows that a healthy diet and exercise help maintain physical health. When pathology sets in, the underlying cause is not always clear. Sometimes it can be hereditary responses to illness, sometimes environmental, and at other times it can be belief systems that create the illness through fear and anger.

While diet and exercise alone are enough to maintain the body, long-term emotional issues can also create disease. Personality traits, such as the over driven 'type A' as documented in the landmark book Reversing Heart Disease by Dean Ornish, M.D., is one example where he documents a man too driven to sustain good heart health. In his studies, he shows that while diet and exercise do help with reversing heart disease, life style changes and emotional stress are also factors. In his heart health program, Dr. Ornish shows that yoga, meditation and peace of mind also play a huge part in supporting a healthy heart and life.

Heart Path can contribute to this both as a form of meditation and as a form of discovering inner peace. Releasing past trauma's and stressors can move a person into greater peace of mind. Allowing for others to be who they are also does the same. Many type A personalities are addicted to extreme control over others. This is a fear-based response. Giving someone tools of self-love helps people come into the moment with more health and vitality.

While most allopathic medicine focuses on the aftermath of heart disease, such as by-pass surgery for clogged arteries, or a pace maker for irregular heart beat, the root cause of illness of the heart is often related to incidents of stress or heart break that are present in a person's life.

Heart Disease

In one recent case, a 58-year-old Latina woman came to me seeking support. She stated that her job was really crazy, working over 60-70 hours a week, her kids were difficult because her youngest son was leaving home and depended on her a great deal and another was dealing with addiction. While she and her husband had a good relationship, he was also very busy and they had little time together. When I scanned her energy field, I perceived all her energy tied in knot around her heart center. While she felt she was being "hit" energetically from all sides, in actuality she was twisting herself around a perfectionist belief "post" inside her heart center. I asked what she wanted most, and she said clearly, "More time with my husband." When I took her into her heart garden, she could see that the belief she had been running was an extreme need to make all people happy and please everyone. Her whole life was twisted around this center 'post' of a demanding inner self. When she was able to perceive the underlying reason for the stress, I suggested she release this belief, and she was gladly able to do so by throwing the 'post' into the bon fire. It was as if the belief was a demanding taskmaster that the fabric of her being was twisted around. I also had her make peace with the aspects that were demanding her to be such a perfectionist. Her mother had died of a heart attack with the same belief running and it literally killed her. When she was able to laugh at herself, "I have tried not to be, but I am just like her." All aspects agreed to let go of this belief and the demands it created. We then had her "separate from her mother's energy by sending both her parents energy back to them, (both were deceased). I could tell she was through the worst of it. Then I took her hands, and without flinching, looked directly into her eyes, and said, "I do not say this often, in fact I cannot remember doing this with anyone else. However, my dear, you MUST take two weeks off immediately! You must go to a beach somewhere, and get horizontal. Do not move, and stay there, let everyone wait on you. Take Dean Ornish's book with you, and begin a new diet immediately. Exercise only by beach walking and swimming, but do not go into high activity, you are exhausted, and dangerously depleted." She smiled and said that she and her husband had planned to leave in two days for Hawaii, without her grown children. I encouraged her to rest before going. "Do not return to work, just take the time off. You have to restore your energy. You are very close to having a heart attack and if you don't rest, and release all responsibility for a time, and then make some serious life changes, you may not be able to enjoy much more of your life with your husband!" She heard my warning.

Three months later she came in, and said that she had decided to retire early, and that her son had moved out, and she and her husband had taken my advice. They reset their priorities, she changed her diet, and released the major stressors in her life. She had also decided to begin a painting class, something she had wanted to do for a long time. Her energy was completely different and was much more balanced, etc. She was using the heart garden to check in with her inner family regularly and she had begun to meditate with the heart garden daily. She had lost some weight, and her heart stress indicators, including high blood pressure, and boarder-line diabetes, had become normalized again, and she was in a much better disposition all the way around. The one session we had together helped her change her life.

Chronic Fatigue

Chronic Fatigue is a difficult and controversial long-term illness that is often mis-diagnosed as multiple sclerosis, or other illnesses. I see this illness on a sliding scale with other immune disorders. Often in discussing life-styles with clients, they indicated extreme perfectionist tendencies with a huge and demanding schedule that kept them running 24/7. The chronic fatigue made them stop and slow down.

In one case of a 45-year-old woman, the pain in her muscles and joints were constant. Over time I was able to help her see that her illness actually was helping her rebalance herself. She began to read more, and support a less stressful lifestyle that included work, but also included play, relaxation, and time with her family. When she delved further, the abuse she had received as a child from her father, was also a factor that she had to release. While I was not the only therapist working with her, she also had a therapist and massage therapist, she said that the sessions we did helped her lift and release patterns of relating with her self that were extremely toxic. Her disease symptoms were reduced and she was able to live in a less demanding way internally. She also got in touch with her spirit guides who brought about a change of relating to herself, and she has been in much better shape physically, mentally, emotionally and spiritually. She now used the illness as an indicator of when she was over doing it.

Cancer

Tumors can be reduced with the Heart Path Process also. This includes malignant tumors. In one case of a 63-year-old mixed-race male, he came in with a diagnosis of prostate cancer. Now this cancer was in very early stages. While he had been a client for sometime, this was a new situation. He was quite upset, as he had just received the news, but he felt it had to do with his history especially on his father's side. As I scanned his system, I found a red dot in his prostate. It was like a red light. When I discussed what I saw, he was willing to go into the heart garden and deal with it. As he went into to the garden and gathered his inner family, I had him bring the energy of the cancer to the outside of his heart garden. He was exhibiting fear through sweat beading on his forehead, and erratic breathing. (The room temperature was actually cool.) When he saw the energy, he sent it love, and it uncoiled into a dragon-like energy. In this experience for both of us, it was related to his father's and grandfather's past in the service in the military—the dragon was both symbolic and literal, as the sign of his grandfather's clan was a black dragon. As he sent the dragon love, it disappeared into the Earth. I then had him look at his family contract. There was a black ribbon tied onto it, and when he released the ribbon, it had the seal of the black dragon. It was as though his family had agreed for future generations to be warriors. He did not want this in his life and wanted to end the "karma." So I had him burn the ribbon, and write the word "complete" on the contract. Then I asked him to call forth his grandfather and his father, and show that the contract had been completed. They released him from further service, and we released the ties between them that bound them to the service of death through war. He then sent it back to the place of records in the etheric realms (Akashic records are an etheric library where all records of life on Earth are kept.) When he did this he felt released from the karma. In the meantime, that red light bulb in his prostate disappeared. He came in for two subsequent sessions where he wanted to make sure this contract was over and the energy reversed. While there were some additional agreements he had to make with himself and his son, there was no more indication of disease.

When he went in for his next test to see his doctor, he reported the cancer markers in his blood work were normal and there was no more indication of the disease. He attributed it to the work we did around his family contracts and the Heart Garden work.

Tumors

In another case, a 48-year-old Japanese American woman came in with a diagnosis of 4th stage lung cancer. When I heard of her illness, a part of me thought I should prepare her for her crossing. But as I spoke to her, it was clear that she wanted to live more than anything. So I began to work with her over a period of months. When she first came to me in April, her breathing was difficult and she had developed a cough. Her coloring was grayish and her energy was low. Honestly I did not think she would last a month in her condition.

In half hour sessions over a period of 6 months every other week she came to me for healing. While we did some guided imagery, and discovered some anger issues, we often worked at releasing her anger at her husband and sons. I used hands-on healing, energy work, and helped her speak to her husband about the way he treated her, as he was extremely emotionally dismissive and hurtful towards her. She had never before said anything except to defend herself, which was fruitless. I encouraged her to speak up about how it felt. She did not engage him in an angry way, but asked him if he wanted to help her. Yes he did she reported. Then she said, "When you put me down it makes me want to leave here. It doesn't help me. Please stop." It only took a few more times of her repeating, calmly her truth, and he stopped! Since I started seeing her, and since money issues were a factor for her, she began to seek free or nearly free support closer to home through Dr. Sha's methods. She still comes in and as of this writing her color is better, her breathing is less labored and she still has a cough. While she is under no illusion about her health, she has more energy and is less anxiety about her situation.

The problem with many clients is that while one can attribute much of the healing to the work I have done with others, it is the willingness of the client to change their patterns of relating with themselves and their past as well as current relationships that makes a lasting difference. In addition, many of my clients, when in a crisis, try anything and everything to reverse their situation including acupuncture, chiropractic, massage, diet, exercise, and other complimentary medicine practices. Some are in therapy, many under the care of a physician. My feeling is that sometimes a combination of things works. Sometimes one leads to more healing than other modalities. Certainly it is clear that extreme stress creates unhealthy people. This has been proven to be the case through studies and books on the topic since the 1980's.[21] Some stress is necessary for vitality, but extreme stress is not good and does not help anything and actually creates disease as many of these studies and books will document. Another book that has a great deal of information about cancer care is Michael Lerner's work *Choices in Healing, Integrating the Best of Conventional and Complementary Approaches,* which you can obtain through the internet through Commonweal-Cancer Help Program in Bolinas, CA. (I worked there for three years as a massage therapist for the program.) This book gives an overview of many cancer modalities and has helped the healing of many facing difficult choices in health care after getting a diagnosis of cancer. His work was documented

---

21   Some sources for reducing stress are: Lawlis, Frank, *Retrain the Brain.* Penguin, 2009: Davis, Martha; Robbins-Eshelman, Elizabeth; *The Relaxation Stress Reduction Workbook.* New Harbinger Publications (1980): Zapolsky, Robert M., *Why Zebra's Don't Get Ulcers.* Henry Holt and Co. (2004)

in the PBS series by Bill Moyers in the 1993 PBS documentary series called, Healing and The Mind, in *The Wounded Healer* segment.

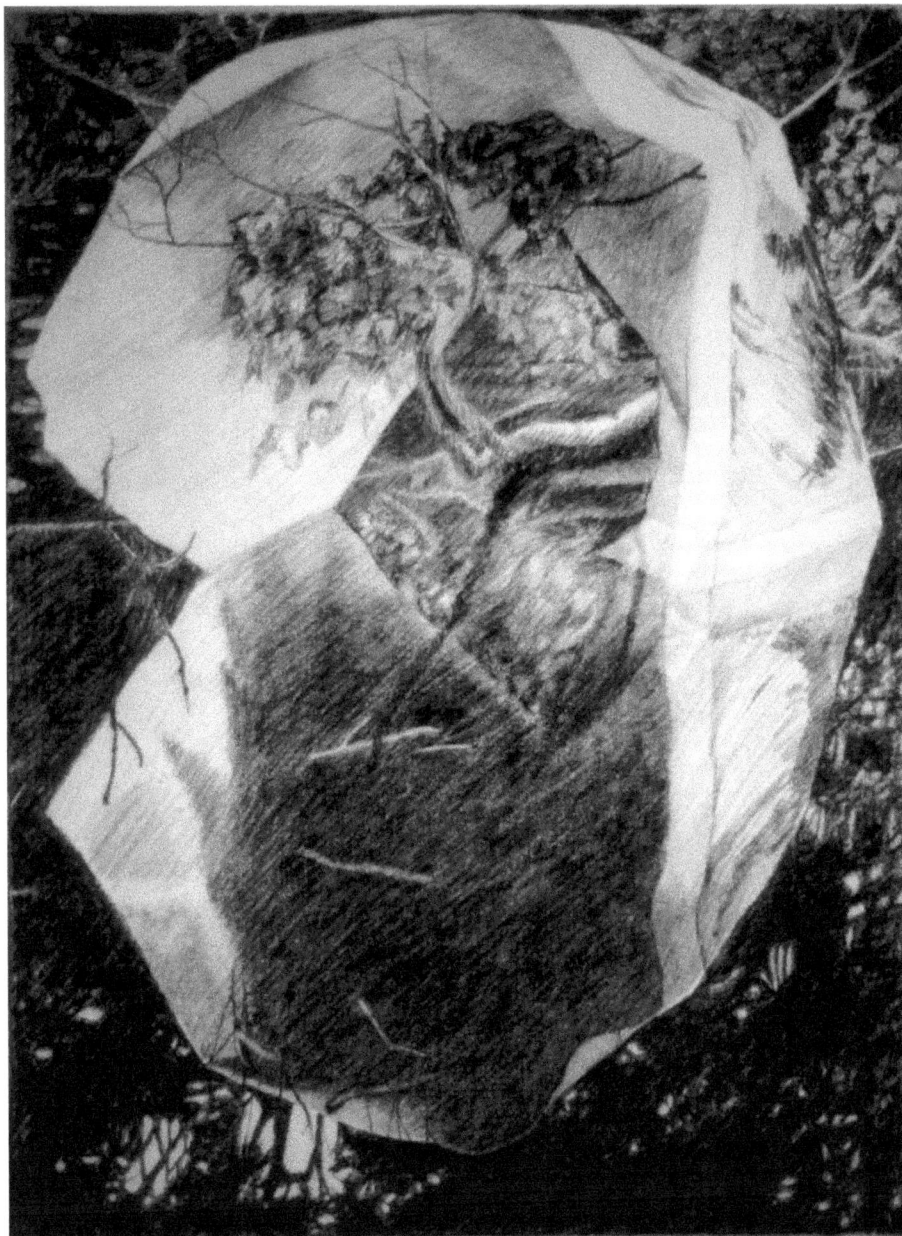

Circle Painting in the Pond -Charcoal on Japanese Paper
by Author

Chapter 4 - Ego Patterns of Relating and their Dynamics

<u>Embrace</u>

First sit silent and feel a hundred hurts.

If you think that's mad,

try sitting still some more

and welcome the hundred swords

that have already pierced your heart.

Notice you are still on the cushion.

Now walk softly and feel the praise begin.

There are a dozens of ways to surrender.

Yet, if you do, before you know it

you are filled with what

you've been looking for forever;

a hundred thousand arms of your own

embracing you.

Negative Patterns of Relating and How to Heal Them - In this section, I would like to delve into ego patterns of relating and how we can discern and dissolve these patterns in ourselves and help our clients as well. I will also address narcissism and self-reflection and why these two concepts need to be 'teased' apart in our understanding. Many people get them confused.

Ego

The Ego is a term first coined by Sigmund Freud to describe three parts of a mental construct that he created. I have inserted my interpretation from a Heart Path perspective in parenthesis. His construct includes the Id, the Ego and the Super-Ego, Id being the instinctual nature (I call this the animal nature), the Ego being the self (what we perceive as the small self), or the 'I' that negotiates between the Super-Ego and the Id, Super-Ego being the unconscious (hidden patterns, belief systems, or operational patterns from which we act).[22] While these three constructs have been widely accepted in psychology as a model of the human mind, they are not really related to the body. They do not include the observer or the higher self. Heart Path relates to the body and the brain or as many psychologist and body workers say, body/mind. It relates to those neuro-pathways that we develop in the body as auto-responses, and it gives a person a way to release those old patterns that are commonly referred to as fight or flight. It also gives people a gentle, compassionate way to release them without judgment. They can be released through loving observation of the inner family. When we love fear-based, or anger-based reactions or constructs we replace those constructs with love, and there is no self-hating or self-loathing mechanism left. It simply dissolves.

It is important to note that some mechanisms are part of the person's make-up. For example, I have a client whose basic nature is one of nervousness. This woman, 65 years old, often fidgets with her hands. (She came in for concern about her husband who was ill.) In one session, as we did the Heart Garden process, we were able to recognize that her main protector inside her heart garden was a squirrel. There was no animal protection for her, her animal protection was prey! When I asked her to bring in other animals, ones that were more predatory, her 'squirrel' grew nervous, but then, quieted down as I suggested that the other predators were there to protect the squirrel. She brought in a mountain lion and a bear (a profound animal of healing in Native American practices and Chinese medicine.) (Besides, they don't generally eat squirrels, I told her.) I noticed more confidence emanating from her,

---

22   Snowden, Ruth (2006). *Teach Yourself Freud*. McGraw-Hill. pp. 105-107. ISBN 9780071472746

but that basic nature is what it is and probably won't change until she gets used to the bear and the mountain lion. It will completely transform as the 'squirrel' surrenders to the higher self and her identity changes from fear to love. In the meantime, she was able to be calmer around her husband, which helped their relationship a great deal.

My definition of ego is the over *inflated, or deflated* self as it relates to the smaller self and bigger Self-described in the introduction as unconditional loving Self (page 10-15). Another way to describe the ego is to say *those aspects that try to control, manipulate or are otherwise un-loving toward the self and others either consciously or unconsciously.* Those aspects that stay in judgment, compare, or go into criticism of one's self or others are ego-based. The 37-year-old male I mentioned earlier is one example. Staying neutral and being with harmony of self and being unconditionally-loving is the key to dissolving the self into Self. Through the Heart Path process a person has a way to slow down enough to observe these mechanisms. They can see them through the various archetypes that play out the dramas of their lives. An example is a child aspect that is trying to run the life of the adult. This happens frequently in alcoholic families. Often when a parent is dysfunctional, a child growing up in that household has to take over certain adult duties before they are ready to assume such responsibilities. They often do not have a childhood. When this happens the child might form beliefs such as "I have to do it myself" or "No one is here for me."

To further clarify, I would say that the ego builds one up or puts one down. It is rarely neutral with those inner messages. Often those messages live unconsciously (Freud's Super-Ego) from past messages from family. Sometimes they are beliefs we formed from childhood or past lives. Beliefs in children form despite a parent's best efforts. Children form beliefs from messages that parents' often mean to be loving, protective or out of their concern for their children. Critical parents often imprint messages that can be destructive to the child. Sometimes a child's inner sense of justice gets ignited with criticism and sometimes they feel oppressed. In any case, messages to the self such as "I'm not enough, or "I am the greatest" have equal impact internally whether given to the child by parents, or created by the child in the course of their growing up.

When you begin to delve into the patterns of the ego in the nervous system, these patterns are "viewed" psychically as machine-like mechanisms, latex or rubbery substances, wiring or blocks. There is a visual 'feel' when you perceive them. Often the patterns are not viewed but felt or perceived by the client or person witnessing the self.

Sometimes I use theatre, comedy, or other devices to "break" the grip of the ego. For example, using a heart garden bon-fire one can release anything--any pattern, or perception or belief no longer needed--into the fire. This releases and transforms the energy. If the "latex" is not dissolving fast enough for my time together with a client, I might suggest loving that pattern into dissolving by sending it love or "painting" pink over the "latex". Sometimes it can be brought into the heart and released into the fire. Often the client does not want to bring the pattern into the heart, which is why other ways of dissolving it outside the garden of the heart works as well. They usually recognize it as un-loving and do not want that pattern in themselves any longer.

The ego patterns create fear, depression, anxiety and they are the underlying cause for some pathology and disharmony. Certainly there are other reasons for pathology, though we do not fully understand the purpose of all illness. Sometimes inherited chemical imbalances such as in depression or in bi-polar disorder are the root cause. Sometimes inherited diseases such as heart disease, or cancers, or other illnesses do not come from our minds or spirits. There is much concern today about environmental illnesses that are caused by pesticides, chemicals dumped on the land, or other environmental pollutants. However, I have found that more times than not, there are some kind of underlying pattern for the disease. In the case of cancers, it can be extreme anger or stress preceding the disease that prompts the illness. Often when someone comes in with a diagnosis from a doctor, I ask them what happened prior to the illness. Many times I have found extreme stress, such as deaths in the family, or eruptions between family members.

In one case of a 72-year-old Caucasian man had a series of deaths, followed by an eruption in trust with a brother over money. A year later, his thyroid was in hyperthyroid mode producing an over-abundance of the hormone thyroxine. There was no family history of the illness. He had radiation therapy and still it was over producing thyroxine. In one conversation, we discovered that all these traumas and losses had occurred starting from two years before the on-set of symptoms. As we talked about what had happened prior to his diagnosis, he reported much regret and lack of forgiveness of the self, unresolved emotions all unexpressed and stuck in the throat. As he released the regrets and grief, I could perceive a black cloud lift from his throat. I suggest he keep writing to release other unexpressed emotions. The results of his tests are not known as of this writing, but he had decided not to repeat the radiation treatment. He felt much better after our conversation. (We did not do the heart garden in this case.)

Sometimes people are carrying chronic diseases to help their families. In one case, a 42-year-old Caucasian woman came in to see me in a wheel chair. She had multiple sclerosis (M.S.). She could only move her head and nothing else. Her body was strapped in and she had a full-time attendant. Her head was strapped in because she had no strength in her neck left. There was a blow tube that she used to move her herself around from one place to the other. As she told me her story, how she had just left her verbally abusive husband, how her mother and grandmother had M.S. and it seemed to be hereditary, how she was able to get her own house so she could spend her last days in peace and give the example to her daughter that she was not going to allow this kind of abuse to continue, how she had gone blind for two years then her sight returned, how her daughter was angry and afraid of getting it and was suicidal, I felt my heart break open with compassion. Then she asked if I could help her to understand why she had this disease, and why it was killing her. I took a deep breath and said that I wish I could snap my fingers and have this disappear, but that I had to be honest and say I didn't think I could help her body. However, I agreed to see what I could get to uncover the reason for this in her karma, if there was an underlying cause. Her spirit may have answers for us. As I looked at her energy field, I was over come by her radiant light. She was a living Bodhisattva, or Divine Being. By her very presence on the planet, she was healing karma, disease, and emotional challenges in her family and in the world. I saw a flame that engulfed her entire body. There were a legion of beings around her, and she was surrounded entirely in golden flames. I had seen the same on Buddhist prayer tankas or sacred paintings. She was burning off and releasing so much, it moved me to tears. When I told her what I saw, her attendant nodded in agreement. He perceived it too. I told her I should be paying her to sit at her feet! In any case, she disagreed and said that she could die in peace now, and felt assured that she had a purpose on earth, despite the conflict and difficulty her family had gone through. She was carrying this disease to help others that was clear enough for her, her attendant and me. I told her I would pray for her daughter and she said she had her seeing a counselor. I will never forget my experience. She was ego-less, entirely embodied as Divine Love.

In the case of ego patterns, the irony is that these patterns are often based on ideas that there is a need for protection, or that the ego is trying to help out or protect the person. The person becomes wrapped in and mired in these protective devices and they become entrapped in the labyrinth of their own minds, hence the small self.

At this point I would like to further define self. While I have already stated that self is the aspect of ourselves that relates to the ego, or that which inflates or deflates us, while the Self is the unconditionally loving and accepting aspect, the small 's' self also relates to our false identities and who we think ourselves to be. Again, this can be positive and negative. As we identify ourselves in jobs, roles, careers, or families, we form a sense of who we are. Our personalities, our character all are aspects of self. But when we identify ourselves as light, or as the love of the Universe, we have a sense of being one with All-There-Is. We still might be in the other roles, but we do not identify with them in the same way as before.

I have had the good fortune to sit with some amazing fully enlightened God-realized beings. (Da Free John or Da Love Ananda, Michael Silverman, Amma, Brenda Morgan, Gurumayi) What was surprising to me, is each had their personality intact. Some examples are how Da was a forceful outpouring of love that bolted through others like lightning. Amma (the hugging guru) emits a wave of love that can be felt for blocks around. What was missing was any need to prove themselves right, any ounce of arrogance, they were serving others with a sense of knowing who they were, but not being boastful about it. However, you could feel the difference in their lack of fear and offering of love openly to anyone.

Here it is important to take a moment to note what the ego does for us. From an Eastern spiritual perspective, the ego defines the small self--which self caught up in the material world. However, we have to have an ego to reach goals in the material world, or to work in positions of power in that world, to discern who one could trust or not trust. Our animal nature, our fight or flight reflexes are part of embodied patterns that we can transform. This paradox is a complex one that many people who are spiritual and living in the ordinary world struggle with. Yet, when an ego is surrendered to Divine Will, to the Cosmic Will, that is love, the ego becomes surrendered in God. There is no conflict. When we surrender our fears to love, we are surrendering our small self to our larger Divine Self. We are living from love rather than fear. While we do not totally drop our reflexive patterns, we are less likely to react from fear and witness and discern what is actually happening in a situation perceived to be potentially dangerous. If there is a sudden attach, such as a loose dog or an aggressive person, those instant reflexes from the animal nature are still there. However a person transformed with love is less likely to attract those situations that require animal instinct.

Peter A. Levine, Ph.D., the leading expert today in trauma therapies, describes this well in his landmark book, *In an Unspoken Voice*, which discusses the fight or flight reactions in humans, and how we, as therapists or healers can work with clients. He recognizes the body maintaining a wisdom all it's own when in true danger. He describes patients he has worked with, with post-traumatic stress syndrome (P.T.S.D.). In understanding the body/mind and brain (brain-stem, animal nature) he shows how trauma can be released in a therapeutic setting through bodily shaking (resetting the nervous system) and allowing the body to do what it needs to do in response to traumatic situations. [23] I found this work very helpful.

When working with clients in the Heart Path process, I find identifying the natural tendencies

of their animal nature helps a great deal in understanding the self. (example the woman with

the squirrel as protection, page 91.) When in relationship with others, it helps a great deal

because if one person in a marriage is a lion in their fight or flight, and another a deer, the

dynamics of the chase or flight can be difficult for both parties. The deer often runs away or

looses when the lion roars and attacks.

Sri Aurobindo, a spiritual and political leader spoke of a new person emerging that is

living in the world as a fully Self-Realized being who surrenders to the Divine Self moment to

moment.

"The supramental transformation means the birth of a new individual fully formed
by the supramental power, the same power that enabled the universe to be created in the
first place from out of a Divine Source. Such individuals would be the forerunners of a new
truth-consciousness based supra-humanity. Among their capacities are: a total oneness
and identity with the environment and with others; total integral knowledge replacing our
essential ignorance, i.e. knowledge by identity; a unification of knowledge and will (what one
knows is automatically created, what is willed is fully known in its truth); the Force of creation
reunited with the Consciousness; and a complete unity of the Individual, Universal, and
Transcendent purpose expressed through the person. Also, all aspects of division and ignorance
of consciousness at the vital and mental levels would be overcome, replaced with a unity of
consciousness at every plane, and even the physical body transformed and divinised. A new
supramental species would then emerge, living a supramental, gnostic, divine life on earth.[24]

He and his companion who he called Mother, laid the foundation for a center in India

dedicated to this end that she carried out for many years after his death. Surely we have not

all evolved to this state, but it is heartening to know that as we work on ourselves and heal

the past we are evolving towards a more expanded consciousness.

Mental pathology is often a deepening of fear/anger patterns until the nervous

system is embedded in these patterns and they become fixed. In addition, I have witnessed

chemical imbalances, and the soul of the person choosing the experiences of say, a bi-polar

23 Levine, Peter, A. *In an Unspoken Voice, How the Body Releases Trauma and Restores Goodness,* North
Atlantic Books, Berkeley, CA, 2010, Chapters 1-7, pages 3-133.
24   Sri Aurobindo, *The Life Divine,* Sri Aurobindo Ashram Trust, Dehli, India, 1977, book II ch.27-

disorder to explore different levels of awareness. However, when pathology appears there can be many related causes including chemical imbalances, hereditary factors, family dysfunction, etc., as mentioned before. One client I had, who came in at the request of her concerned mother, was a 37-year-old mother of three. The client admitted to me that she liked the highs and lows of her disorder. She did not want to change a thing either with medication or any other sort of treatment. In the case of this client, she was exploring the pathway of the bi-polar state, she had a husband willing to help her when her state got too erratic. Who was I to interfere with her exploration or their karma?

Many of us to some extent have these patterns when we are imbalanced. My perception is that some have their root in the ego, some in the physical, some come as lessons of the spirit, and some are imbedded patterns of behavior. What we believe and experience can make a difference when it comes to the chemical imbalances. It is important to understanding how the ego gets entrenched in certain tracks of thinking that do us no good and how we might release them. Heart Path can help release trauma.

In cases of sever trauma those 'trauma vortexes" or the 'fear/immobility cycle'[25] we become energetically frozen and our protective nature begins to isolate from the rest of the self or in extreme cases paralyses the client. In Peter Levine's book, *Waking the Tiger*, and *In an Unspoken Voice*, he describes these areas of trauma in the brain through the vagus nerves[26] and how they function. [25] He states:

Most people think of trauma as a "mental" problem, even as a 'brain disorder." However, trauma is something that also happens in the body. We become scared stiff or, alternately, we collapse, overwhelmed and defeated with helpless dread. Either way, trauma defeats life. ...The indigenous people throughout South America and Mesoamerica have long understood both the nature of fear and the essence of trauma. What's more, they seem to know how to transform it through their shamanic rituals. ...(In) Shamanic traditions, where healer and the sufferer join together to re-experience the terror while calling on cosmic forces to release the grip of the demons. The shaman is always first initiated, via a profound encounter with his own helplessness and feeling of being shattered, prior to assuming the mantel of healer. Such preparation might suggest a model whereby contemporary therapists

---

25   Levine, Peter, *In an Unspoken Voice, How the Body Releases Trauma and Restores Goodness*, North Atlantic Books, Berkeley, CA, pages 21-22.
26   Ibid, pages 18-20 illustrations.

must first recognize and engage with their own traumas and emotional wounds. [27]

My personal experience with clients and within my own inner work is that for some, these traumas are mitigated with Heart Path. As we go into the Heart Garden with the client, we are drawing on our own work with ourselves and on our experiences with others in sessions, not to mention our training as healers. People with severe trauma--due to horrific abuse or other root causes--may need the help of a trained psychotherapist who works with these patterns on a regular basis to mend the person's psyche. However, I find that much healing can take place with Heart Path and it can be used as a tool for this kind of work by many different sorts of people involved in healing and many different kinds of trauma. The disembodied soul loss often returns when called back with love and no judgment.

I have done work with women and men in jail who were diagnosed as schizophrenic and it worked well enough to help them see the pattern of their behaviors and assisted them in integrating some of their 'voices'. In one case, a 35-year-old woman was wounded by incest when she was a child. She turned to prostitution to make her living, which is an all too common pattern in society. Though my time with her was severely limited due to restrictions with the jail system, in just three half-hour sessions, she did get some relief. We were able to integrate some of her voices, as she recognized them as aspects of herself. She reported relief from the most critical ones, with a lessening of their impact on her. She also grew bored and sick of her life-style and was willing to look at some life changing ways away from prostitution and towards a legitimate living.

Several other jail clients began to look more consciously at their behaviors. They also began to release some of these aspects and integrated them in some group work that we did. The aspects described as 'voices' were parts of themselves that were split off and not helpful to them. They usually had derogatory messages that were begun when the client was very small with some sort of traumatic incident. Other times the client's behavior in drug and

27   Levine, Peter A. *In an Unspoken Voice, How the Body Releases Trauma and Restores Goodness*, North Atlantic Books, Berkeley, CA. pages 31-35

alcohol dependencies or risky behaviors on the streets were what set parts to disassociate after the initial wound. Rape and incest were common themes. When one is able to create a safe internal and neutral place in one's self, the patterns can be seen and reconciliation occurs within the psyche. The person feels more whole and at peace.

There are many such ego patterns of thinking. For example, there is much in the psychological media about narcissistic behavior, and how to recognize it. There is no doubt that narcissism is how a person's ego pattern draws others around them to support the illusion of their grandiose self. This is part of a pathology that harms others in the process, as the narcissist does not care really about the consequences for others, resulting from their behavior. All they know is how they "need" what they 'need" and will do anything to get it no matter how harmful.[28]

However, there is a great difference between narcissism, self-inquiry or self-reflection, and witnessing, and often people, clients and therapists in pop-psychology confuse them. While narcissism is a destructive pattern, self-inquiry and self-reflection are part of a contemplative process that brings about confrontation of the self in the reality of the present moment. It brings the parts from the past into current time. The person practicing self-inquiry develops the observer within or the witness self. It is a path that leads to ego dissolution and transformation. Like Heart Path it gives the person a way to witness their patterns of relating. Heart Path helps the process with love and compassionate observation. In fact, any form of meditation will help, but Heart Path is 'targeted' on healing the self into Self.

The 'self' into the Self

As described before and throughout this text, the small self dissolves when the larger Self, or unconditional loving Self, is allowed to be. Often I find that as these entrenched patterns dissolve with the Heart Path process. The person moves from valuing 'doing' *over* 'being', to valuing 'being *with* doing.' In our Western culture, we are so driven to achieve and produce that the 'being' nature, or the feminine nature, the feeling aspect of a person, and the higher Self—a person's presence—is not often recognized or valued. Heart Path supports this shift of consciousness. As humanity comes into more awareness of 'being *with* doing' the masculine (doing nature) has to begin to serve the 'being', rather than dominate it. Domination and control issues are ego-driven. The feminine nature can also be dominating and emotionally controlling, so the pattern can exist on either side of the person. However, when the patterns dissolve the person evolves. This is how evolution of our species is occurring today. It is very exciting to witness.

Patterns of Relating and Witnessing Them

There are many patterns in relating that are unhealthy for love to simply be expressed without negativity. All one has to do is think of popular songs that speak of love going wrong to see the myriad of ways that we limit love's expression. Some of the song lyrics refer to patterns of possessing the other such as, "can't live without you," "don't want to live if living is without you," from the Bee Gees along with other dramatic lyrics are examples. All of them are exhibiting unhealthy patterns of dependence and difficult ways to create love relationships. Just witnessing these patterns can help bring them to consciousness and dissolve them. Of course, the aspects of self have to agree to try something new.

The most common pattern of ego relating is the **victim-perpetrator pattern**, or master-slave, which much of our culture, including the media, loves to go on about. It is a very limited and toxic pattern of relating. It only allows for one polarized relational ping-pong way of viewing another. If one is the victim, you must be the perpetrator, if you become the victim everyone else is the perpetrator. However, there are so many other ways of relating having nothing to do with victim-perpetrator. Many of them are quite pleasant and wonderful. One must be willing to give up the drama of relating in this manner. Once you stop playing the games, people shift and relating changes.

There are several other patterns of the ego, which get imbedded into the system. Usually they can be a sign of a fear-based reality or an anger-based reality. Many of them will be presented as one or the other. I will go into various ego-patterns of relating and how the client in the therapeutic setting can witness them.

The first reality that anyone offering healing assistance must come to terms with is: Does the person before me really want to heal? If the answer is no, then there is nothing one can do and the person needing help has limited their capacity to transform. If the answer is yes, then there is hope and anything can be shifted, recognized and healed.

How does one dissolve such patterns? By recognizing the behaviors, we can change them; sometimes the underlying pattern will still be there to 'return to, just in case.' Releasing the patterns altogether through Heart Path make a person more loving and less critical of oneself and others. Bringing the pattern to the front of the heart garden and witnessing it, or witnessing it inside the heart garden, dissolves it as we witness with our true nature, the unconditionally loving self. When one releases these patterns in one's self it helps others to let them go, too. There seems to be a critical mass, where the culture releases the pattern as more and more are empowered to do so. I will discuss more on this micro-cosmic/macro-cosmic effect later in the book. First let us look at these patterns and then I will share how they get released with Heart Path.

Having to always be right

Often a fear of being wrong demands that we must always be right. Anyone participating in the EST training from the 80's has been confronted with this pattern of relating to others. This pattern gets associated with 'good and bad' or 'I am right and therefore good, and you are wrong and therefore bad.' It is also presented in angry lashing out when others are right and the other one is proven 'wrong.' To get one's way often leads to self-destructive ways or self-limiting behavior wrapped around the pattern of being right. Once a person realized they don't have to be right, it frees one from the fear of making mistakes.

I remember attending the EST seminars years ago in Michigan in the 1980's. The release of energy in me of 'not having to be right' was an amazing experience. I didn't have to continually prove myself. I noticed that others had similar reactions. As the training was held all over the country, it helped to release a pattern in the collective ego that was restraining our culture. While there are plenty of people who still need to be right, as witnessed by our political system, many now recognize the pattern in others and in the self more readily than 20 years ago.

Manipulation and Lying

Associated with having to be right are often patterns of manipulating others and lying about what happened to get one's way. Disrespect and making others wrong are some of those methods. A person with this pattern embedded will lie and have no real consciousness about the pattern.

Control

Everyone needs to have control of their personal environment and their way of being in order to have self-identity. However, extreme control issues are based on fear of being out of control. Some folks want to control everything and everyone around them. This can prevent one from going with the flow of their life force. There can also arise with the release of a particular fear, that is, a fear of being with *what is*. As we evolve and release fear, the one surrendering releases extreme control of others and everything around them and the self is transformed into Self (fear to love).

Mind Games

These are usually "check/check-mate" ways that trap others into a web of convoluted thinking. Often mind-games are used by men and women to trap or confuse their victims. Yes, you guessed it! This is another victim/perpetrator pattern variation. Often the person playing the mind games is trapped in there with the one being 'played'. Since the one playing the games are making the 'rules' they are in control. They exert their control with destructive notes, usually anger, fear or a combination. These ways often force the other person into confusion and keep others off balance. This can be a deadly game of cat and mouse.

The trouble is life itself can be viewed as a game. Often we are playing games constantly in our work, in our lives and in our education. These can be fun and can help us find our sense of self. However, mind games draw energy away from the normal activities of the day and we get our energy caught up in whatever the mind game is. We become enmeshed in someone else's thinking patterns, or worse, our own. To break these patterns, they need to be seen for what they are. They need to be viewed in the light of consciousness and with a little objectivity. Sometimes just calling them what they are—mind games—stops the pattern. They are based on power-over another, rather than power-with, and have little to do with evolution. One way to use the Heart Garden process for this is to bring the pattern to the outside the heart garden to look at it. Another way is to start with the person playing the game and view the client, or the client's adversary, outside the heart garden gate. You can suggest that they look at the dynamics of relating with another. As your client's presence and your own presence is brought to bear on the pattern, there is a release of the pattern and there is another layer released of self-loathing or distracting behavior.

Compartmentalization

We live in a world with multiple activities, functions and demands on our time. We tend to live in a world with many facets, and there are many facets of ourselves that are expressed that have to respond to those world functions.

Compartmentalization is one response to functioning everyday. It divides up the mind so that there are separate activities that one does expressing different personalities and different characters of us. While not pathological, it is an ego pattern that segments the self. In extreme compartmentalization one thing in a person's life doesn't have anything to do with the other. Split personalities, people with schizophrenia, or multiple personalities are extreme cases. However, we all have ways of compartmentalization that keeps one activity distinct from another to help us focus on the task at hand.

The truth is we are one person, and the compartmentalization pattern is just that, a pattern of disconnection or of duality. It is sometimes a way for us to do what one part of us doesn't like the other part doing. While we are not playing a game, we are in a way dividing our energies and not wanting to admit that the walls we have between things are taking up a lot of energy to maintain, they are being maintained to protect us from guilt, shame, or self-judgment, or judgment from others. The problem with compartmentalization is that when those different parts of our selves meet, it can be like an earthquake. The walls come tumbling down, and we feel exposed. Actually it is a good thing, but it feels devastating and disorientating at first. When a person is very compartmentalized in their thinking, it is often a fear-based way of managing their lives. It often happens when one is having an affair, or when there are several parts of our lives that are in conflict with one another.

While men tend to compartmentalize more than women, it happens in both sexes, and it is not always fun to deal with as a therapist, because the client gets so used to living in separate 'safe' worlds, that when a wall comes down, defenses come up. Sometimes anger, fear or a combination comes up at the therapist. Sometimes there are serious splits in the psyche. People hide so well, that they don't want to be exposed.

In one case, a male friend of mine who was an African-American psychologist and medical doctor had two very distinct personalities to such an extent that he had two clothes closets to express those two people. He could show me the two sets of clothes, but he could not integrate the two personalities within himself, though he was working on it. He was well aware that both aspects provided him with benefits that he could not reconcile. Both judged the other, one being more conventional than the second aspect, and neither of them like the other at all.

Heart Path works well with this configuration because it is less threatening to the ego aspect that devises the walls. If the person can know that it is safe to come out, and create that safety in the heart garden, this pattern can be released. Of course the person that maintains the division has to want to release it. When someone is serious about transforming the ego, there is nowhere to hide and one has only to pay attention to this pattern to let it go. It certainly releases a lot of energy that can be used for other things!

Releasing Patterns of the Ego

With all patterns of the ego, whether victim-perpetrator, manipulation, lying, control, mind games, compartmentalization, or any other pattern one might come across, the way to transform these patterns in the Heart Garden is the same. We first align with the light of our being with the three stars of the self; we then gather the aspects of the self together in the Heart Garden; we witness the pattern outside or inside, depending on the client and where the pattern lies so that the client can look at it; make new decisions about it's usefulness; and we let it go. Forgiveness of the self is crucial to this transformation as well as the forgiveness of others who might have given them this pattern, such as a parent or partner. When the release happens, there is usually a sense of freedom in the client, often times the client is glad to be done. Sometimes the pattern will show up again in other relationships in the inner family. If this happens, often I will ask the client to make a new agreement inside with all of the inner family so that they are free of this pattern once and for all through all time and space. This works very well.

It also goes along with Buddhist and Hindu teachings that center between patterns of duality as a way to transform these patterns. In many of these patterns, the ego is split in a dualistic reality that causes pain of separation. Healing separation is what the Heart Path process is all about. It helps reconcile the duality to create a better, more harmonious inner world that will eventually resonate with the unconditional loving authentic Self.

Past Time and Lives

Past lives are part of present time because everything exists in this moment. Every part of the past is in our energy field. We carry it all around with us. It lives in us until we can release the trauma, memory or challenge of the past.

Once I was working offering readings at a psychic fair. During a lull in the action, a man came up to me with the intention of proving that past lives do not exist. He came with a pendulum in hand and showed me the *yes* and *no* direction of a pendulum he carried. Then he asked the question: *Do past lives exist?* Of course the pendulum moved in the *no* direction. Why? Because he didn't believe in them, and the pendulum moved according to his will. This was how he created proof for himself of being right. I suspect he has some issues with women as well to prove his male superiority.

I found it irritating, especially because my sign to the public said 'past life readings' as well as a list of other services I offered. After controlling my irritation at his obvious ego need to be right and make everyone else wrong, I said to him calmly, "Of course they don't exist in the past, there is no past. There is only the present moment. However, the memory and imprint of those experiences do live on today until we integrate the lessons of the past." He did not like my retort, went on to another psychic to tell them how wrong they were about

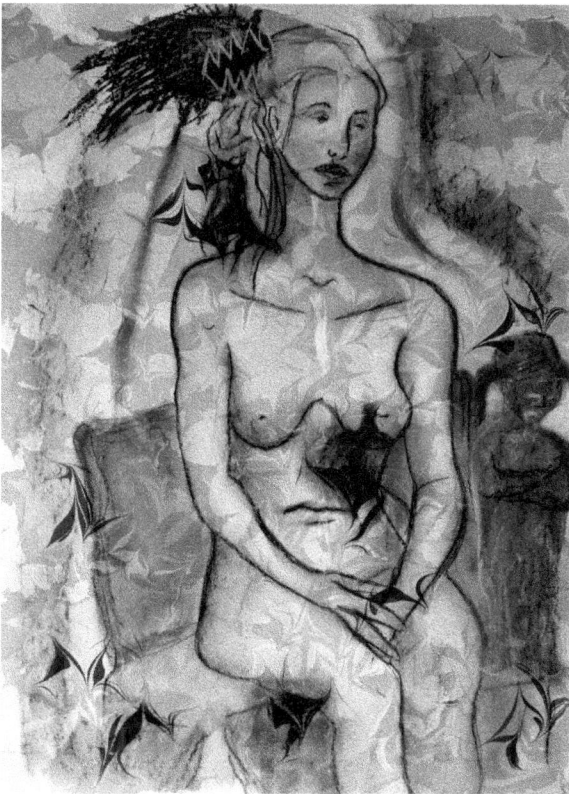

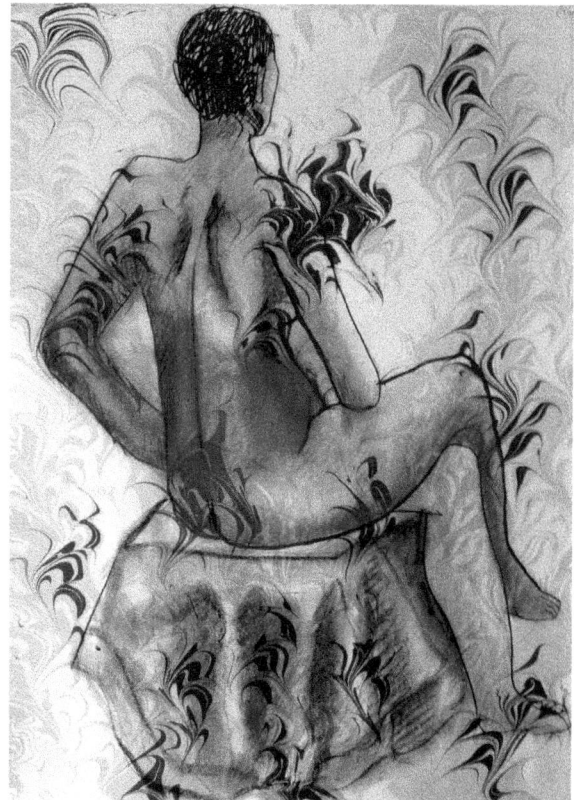

Negative energy stuck in a person with negative spirits

Stuck Anger in tbe third and second chalkra

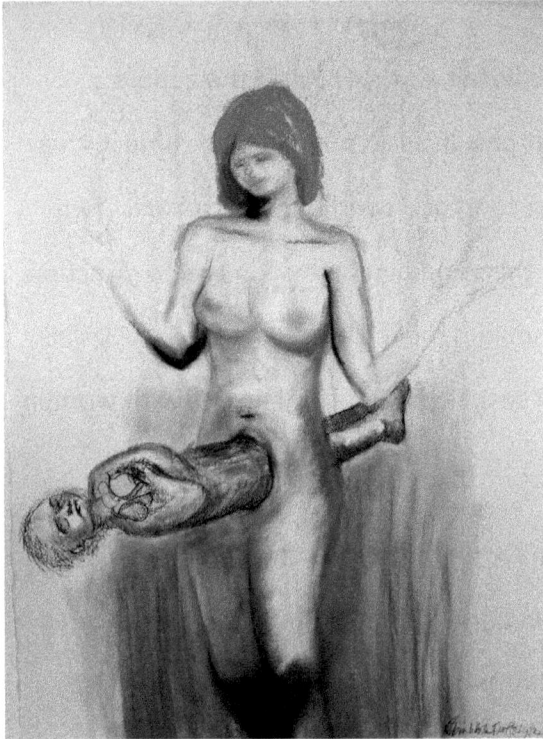

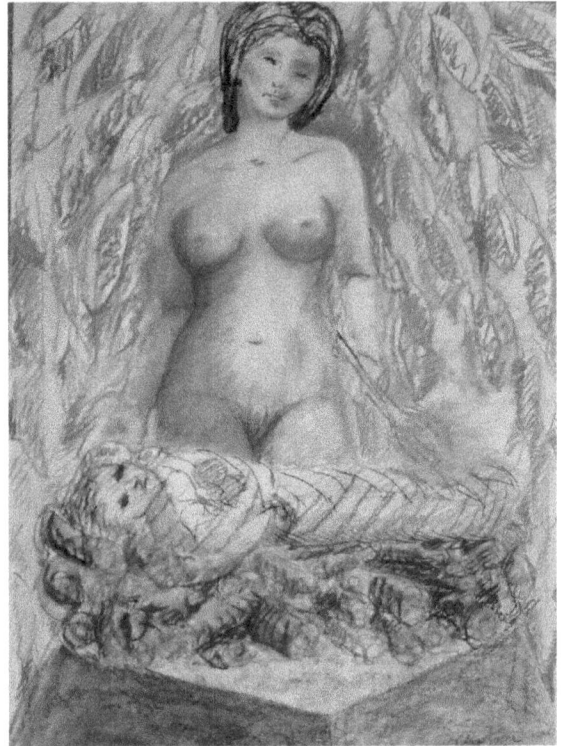

Left: Shows a dead part of the self that has been held in the second chakra.

Right: Response to letting go shows the release in a energetic funeral pyre.

Left: Experience of a client with "holes in the head" from where the client stored lies from others that she believed.   Right: The transformed self to Self.

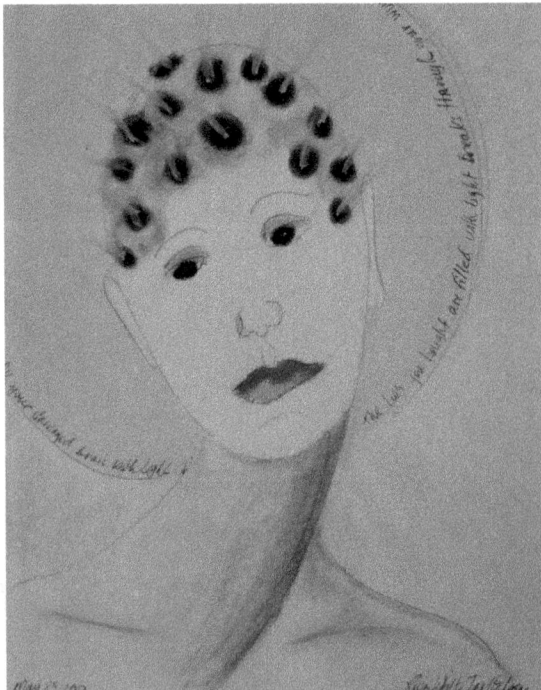

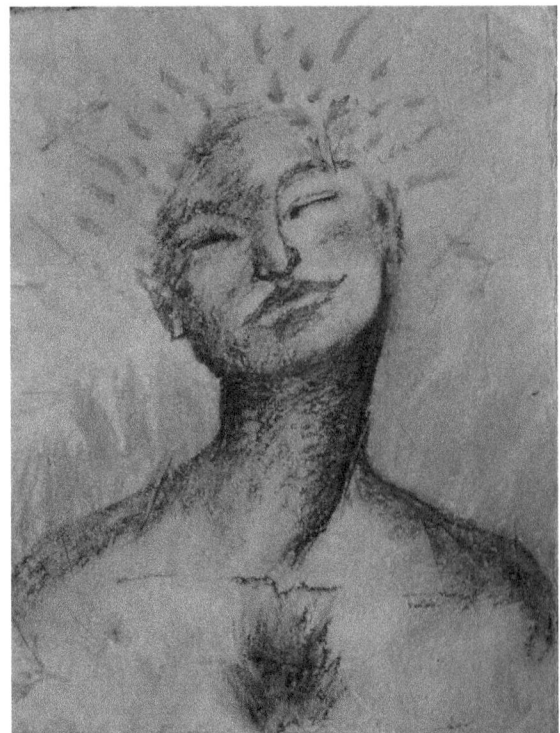

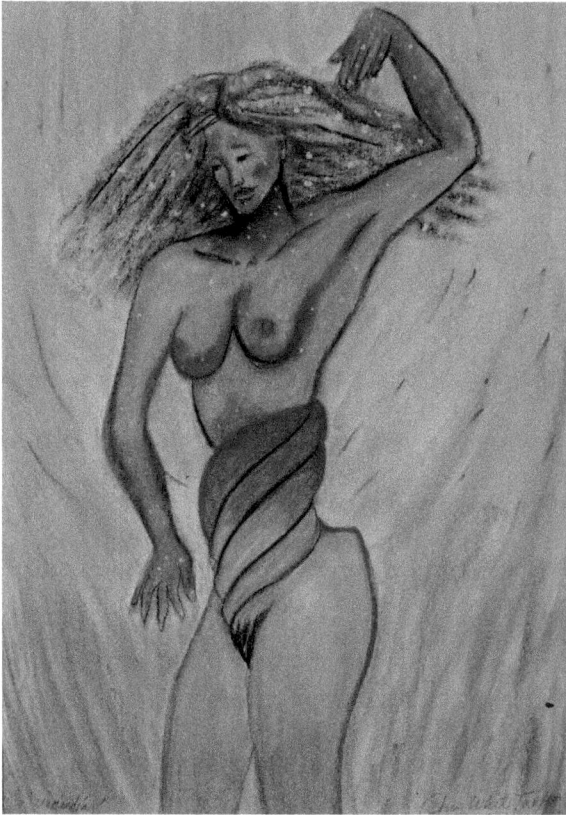

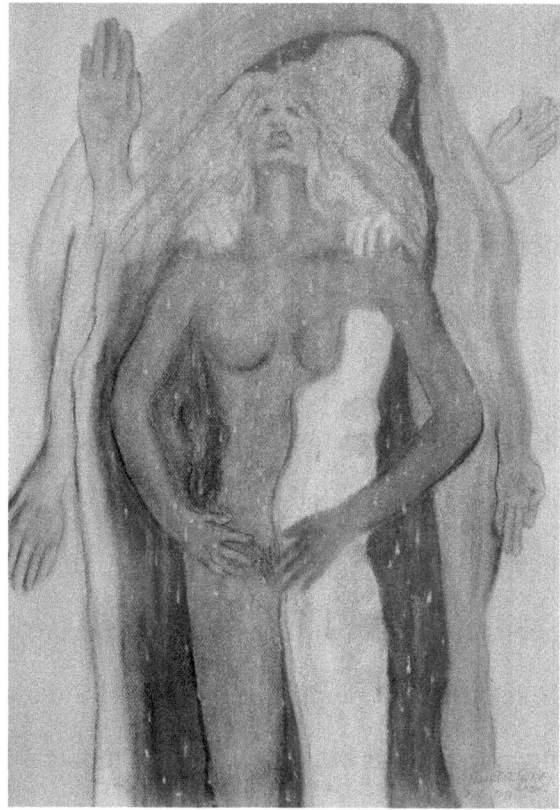

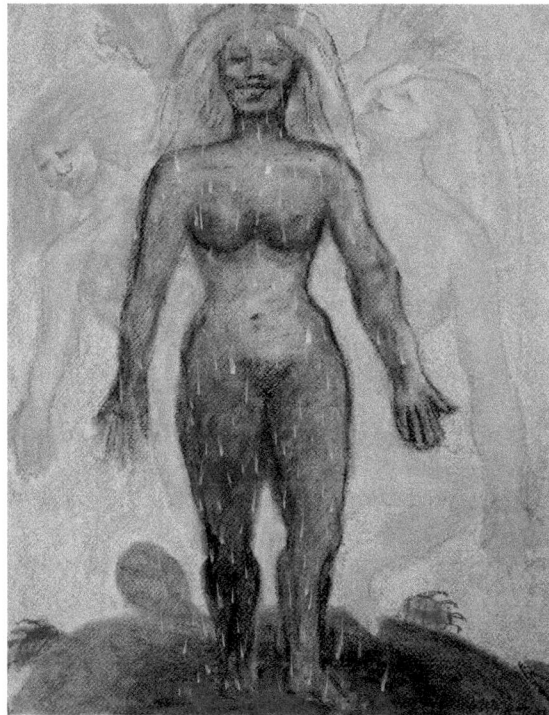

Drawings left to right to bottom: A person "unwinding" in a session from blocked energy in the 2nd chakra. This was not a physical unwinding, but a spiritual one. The person's energy unwound. having been literally 'twisted round oneself' financially, creatively and personally. This action released a paralysis caused by a "cast of fear" worn underneath the twisting in a subsequent session and third drawing shows the release of the "cast of fear" in the system entirely after a third session. This release shows a common ego pattern, that of "freezing with fear" or armoring that I often perceive.

past lives, but thankfully I had another client and moved on.

Everything is in present time, even the past experiences. When a trauma or big event occurs in our existence, no matter how long ago, a part of our selves stays there to witness the lesson, to figure out what happened. This occurs especially if the event was violent. Human history is full of wars and destruction. Our history books are full of these occurrences, in fact very little of history can be discussed without wars and violence at the forefront. Our existence is much bigger than just this one lifetime. We have lived many existences in many forms over the millennia. However, if those lives were lived during war, famine, or other such commonplace occurrences on Mother Earth, we are given an opportunity with Heart Path to release the trauma and integrated the aspects of the past. Those aspects are still trying to figure out what happened. So it is important that they be given the benefit of perspective. Once they receive perspective, it is easier to reconcile the situation and integrate the experience and the energetic aspect that has been left behind. Once integrated, the energy is released and the person is made more whole as a result. The witness in us helps a great deal. Through the witness self, and through the therapists support of the client's energy to face what occurred, we learn the lesson and move on. Those old patterns are reformed and the energy is freed up to use for current life adventures. Often past-life trauma comes up as a result of current lifetime issues, so there is no need to 'go fishing' for such lifetimes. They will occur naturally through traumas in the person's current lives compounded with the added feature of the client's emotional response triggered from the past. This response will appear to be big and out of proportion to the current lifetime challenge. You deal with them the same way as you would a current life issue. It helps to 'clear" and release as much emotion as possible with images of release with the bonfire, or a hot air balloon going up into space taking it away.

Healing the Trauma of Past Lives

Often the very people that played roles as mother, father, brother, sister, lover, in other lifetime with us, are playing out new ones in this lifetime as well. I call it our karmic circle.

We can have several of these over time with different groups of people. The love draws us back to be with each other and to work out what we need to together. When forgiveness is achieved today, it can reach backwards deeply into the past. Drama's today may be reflected in the past, but until the past-lives are addressed complete forgiveness will be difficult to realize. Usually I find that people will come in with an insight that they have history with a person beyond this lifetime. They usually want to find out what happened and what needs to be addressed currently to release the past. They will need to address both the past and their current crisis for a complete release of trauma, most of the time. Again, the wisdom of the client brings up the issue and knows what to heal—they just may not know how to get there.

Sometimes the wound is left but the content is irrelevant. For example, just the other day, I had a client that had a dark pool inside her heart garden. This had never occurred before with any other client. My interpretation was that the 'pool' was full of self-hatred. I asked her how it felt and she confirmed the feeling I perceived. She perceived the pool too, and asked about it. When I had asked the client to send the pool love, her love dried up the 'puddle' and the person did not have any bruising in her heart remaining from the image. Checking in with her afterwards, asking how it felt inside now, she said, "I feel so free!" While this may be quite unconventional, my client could not have talked her way out of that puddle or process it. In order for the pool of self-hate to transform, it needed to be healed with the only thing that does healing and that is love. There was no need to dwell on the fact of what it was. It just needed to dissolve. It could have been in there from past incarnations for a very long time. Just like old family feuds that go on for generations, the original injury is forgotten. Only the bruising remains. Content was not important at that moment, though on another occasion it might have been, what was important was to release it.

When past lives present themselves in a session, or are spoken by the client, there are many ways to handle them. First I ask the client to go into the heart garden, checking in first with all the aspects to; a) make sure all the aspects are working together; and b) to make sure their past life is not present time aspect of the self locked in an inner struggle with another of their aspects. There is a difference between an aspect of the self that is fighting with other aspects, and one that is in battle with another person. It is wise to tease them apart and deal with one at a time. Sometimes this happens when the person has their parents living *as* their adult male or female aspect. To separate these aspects, I ask the parent to leave the adult female, and/or male, and have them witness themselves as they truly are. Thank the parents and let them go to live in their own heart garden.

Then once the inner family is assembled and peacefully living together in the Heart Garden, the masculine and feminine can support each other's needs and are working together. The masculine supporting the feminine or 'doing' supports 'being,' and the 'being' loving the 'doing' aspect; both masculine and feminine parts are caring for and in relation to the child. The higher self is there for everyone and offers wisdom and advice when asked. The child is not in charge of handling emotionally charged situations of the inner family and therefore can feel free to play.

Sometimes I ask the client to bring down a screen in front of their heart garden and see if they can run the old movie of the past life on the screen. Often they will get flashes of costumes, and a scene or scenario. I tune in as well and add what I perceive. This way we might each get pieces of the picture. Again, I make sure to rely on *their* pictures as much as possible, rather than mine, though sometimes if their movie stops or they don't see what happened due to the trauma, and I do, I offer my suggestions. Because it didn't happen to me, I am often able to fill in the blanks of what I perceive for them. Sometimes I get clear pictures of what happened and offer those pictures to them.

In one case of a 35-year-old Latina woman, who was being tormented by neighbors who were in gangs (she wasn't), came in asking to understand what had happened in past lives to cause this kind of antagonism with apparent strangers. As she went into her Heart Garden and brought her inner family together, we brought the screen down in front of the Heart Garden to show her what had happened. As the movie ran, she could perceive a time in a past life where the roles had been reversed. Then the pictures stopped for her. She desperately wanted to continue and understand what had happened. So I looked on the 'other side' of the screen, and could see that she had done some terrorizing herself to them. I reported what I 'saw' and asked if she could forgive herself. As she did, I asked that she bring the person she was from the past forward, by having that aspect step out of the screen. Bringing the suppressed terrorizing aspect to the Heart Garden out of the past, she showed her a movie of her present karma that she had initiated. The person she had been felt remorse, and she was able to integrate the aspect into the Heart Garden with complete forgiveness of her self.

Depending on the client, seeing what traumas there are and what needs to be forgiven makes all the difference in healing. This same woman had walked in like a rag doll, but she walked out as though she had gained a new vitality, her head up, eyes straight and shoulders back, looking radiant.

Sometimes I ask a client to 'fast forward the movie' to conclusion of a past lifetime when they are leaving the body and transitioning into spirit. I ask them to bring that spirit to the front of the heart garden. I ask them to ask the spirit; "What did they learn from that lifetime?" "What is needed?" Can they, a) Forgive the other person? b) Forgive them selves? c) Integrate the part of them from the past that needs to come home to the Heart Garden? When they have accomplished this I move into present time with current relational challenges and proceed as you would to integrate or solve issues.

Sometime, if it is a relationship challenge with a current time relationship, I ask the client to bring the person in conflict to the Heart Garden and have them talk to them, sometimes using a talking stick to referee their conversation. If the other person is extremely negative, I look for cords or other ways they keep the person "tied into them" energetically.

At other times a person just loves high drama, and they are not about to change the dynamics. If this is the case, I point it out and move on. I don't dwell on it. Until a person is ready to drop high drama, there is nothing one can do, short of pointing it out, to change it. For them to notice their drama king or queen is a huge step. Sometimes, if they are tired of high drama, I ask them to just watch it as it arises and see if there are less dramatic reactions or choices available.

There are many other questions you might ask during the process of helping them move to forgiveness, which is always necessary if the person really wants to heal. Some other relevant questions during the process might be; "What happened next?" (Who killed or tortured whom) "How is the relationship today?" "What traces of the past are still operating?" "Do they want to continue relating in this manner?" "How can they change their dynamics?" "Can they see the pattern and how entrenched it is?" "What would work for them to change the pattern?"

Often the trauma of the past feels vague and as though it is of an old movie. This is good! It is easier to forgive when things are not so emotionally charged. Sometimes the client wants to hold on to the wound. Two things work well to move them along towards forgiveness. The first is to ask them; "What are you getting out of holding on to this wound?" The second is to have them look at an older movie where they did the very perpetration to the other person. Sometimes it is easier to see the wounds that we have had inflicted upon us and not so easy to see the wounds that we inflict on others.

When a person has reached forgiveness of the other person and the self for agreeing to be a part of this wounding and lesson, the karma is released. It is important to have the client forgive themselves. "All forgiveness is self-forgiveness," as the Charles and Myrtle Fillmore's 'New Thought,' teaches through Unity Churches, Science of Mind and Religious Science Churches in many of their books[29]. I have found this to be true. When one forgives one's self, one has completed the karmic cycle. It helps us move on.

The last two questions to ask the client are; "Can you forgive them and can you

29   Charles and Myrtle Fillmore, *The Twelve Powers of Man*, Unity Publishers, continuously published without copyright since publication.

forgive yourself?" When the client has examined themselves for the answers, and they come up with 'yes' in both cases, the healing is complete. If they cannot in either case, forgiveness becomes their homework. Often I suggest they go home and write about it to process the whys. Sometimes just sitting with the lack of forgiveness outside the heart garden (while the client is inside the garden) works to dissolve the lack of forgiveness, resentment and trauma of the past.

Energy Medicine and Shamanism

Energy Medicine (EM) is the practice of using energy to help people heal on a physical, emotional, mental or spiritual level. It is in relationship to nature in that it aligns us with our human nature and more deeply connects us with the natural world. The elements of the natural world live through us, and some of us are learning to discern ourselves as integral to nature as air, fire, water or earth, not just on or in those elements. We are those elements. EM is related to natural healing in a long line going back to laying on of hands, and many other forms of healing that some natural healers have practiced over the centuries.

Personally I see EM as connecting people with their authentic selves so that they can better function in this world. In today's world, energy medicine can take the form of guided imagery, energy healing, herbal remedies, massage, acupuncture, chiropractic, cranial-sacral therapy, kinesiology, and many other forms of healing through manipulation of the body, laying new landscapes in the mind, or aligning spiritually with the divine force of love.

When a person sees energies, spirits, and entities, it is no different from perceiving energy that is in a body. It is just energy out of body. Normally in the West, a person with these abilities is called a medium--that is they walk between worlds--there are no barriers to the spirit world. They perceive the spiritual realms. Sometimes this is called shamanism in other cultures. Shamans journey to other spiritual worlds to retrieve information or aspects of the self, to close portals, or help others heal on a soul level. They may use drums and rattles, ceremonial costumes, or they may just sit with a person who is hurting and discern what their realties are energetically.

From these definitions that I have just offered, there is not a lot of difference between one form of working with energy and another in their essence, however the form definitely varies!

In many indigenous cultures, spirits help in the healing of body, mind and emotions, and especially spiritually. People go to ceremonies or Lawampi ceremonies (Lakota tradition) to get messages from the spirits of light who guide them and help them heal. In these ceremonies, as in other indigenous ceremonies, the spirits come in and interact with people who need help. It is an amazing experience. I have attended several Lawampi ceremonies and many other ceremonies in various Native American spiritual traditions, and I find them to be extremely helpful, healing, and unique in what they offer people and how they are created. Most native healers will tell you the form they take comes from their spiritual guidance.

The same can be said for the ceremonies of any shaman. They interact with the natural world to help people with healing. These ceremonies are not manipulating the natural world—they are engaging it. This differs from witchcraft because with the dark arts, there is manipulation of natural energies, which I consider dangerous. Often there is no humility involved and often the danger is the bypassing of free will on the part of the person being effected. There is benevolent "white" witchcraft where healing and humility and a good deal of concern about balance are part of the spells and potions. This is different than the dark arts or black witchcraft. Anytime manipulation is involved you are dealing with the ego, not the surrendered state of being so necessary for humility.

What is important to understand is that all these methods use energy. Energy is neutral and cannot be created or destroyed, though it can change form. This is the basic understanding of Energy Medicine. When you offer guided imagery to a client, you are helping them witness their internal landscape and interact with it. You become the tour guide to the inner world of their body, emotions, mind, and spirit, which demands a lot of objectivity, witnessing, compassion and humility, because we do not have all the answers, none of us do. I find using guided imagery is often surprising and humbling, because I do not find it to be predictable.

Personally I feel that the answers come from within the client I am serving anyway. Most of what I do is mirror back the person's statements so they can hear themselves. This gives me the clues for beginning to address a person's healing needs.

As an example, I had a client recently who had a feeling of being attacked at home, at work, and in her life in general. This was a 43 year-old woman who worked in a business as an executive administrator. She managed many people, and in her home life, she lived with other women in community who wanted to have a conscious community of people to interact with in their shared home. This woman had a history with these roommates in previous lives. As we did more sessions, we could perceive them together. Sometimes I would see an aspect in the shadows, or she would feel that her reactions were bigger than what was happening in her present-time reality. Most of these lives were lived in battle. She had many as a monk, or warrior, where her (him in past lives) first line of defense was to attack.

In this case, I was able to say to her that the world today is not out to get her. But she was still in the victim /perpetrator dynamic where most people were just trying to work things through with her. She got it, that her default pattern was defense, while her present time friends are not calling for such strong reactions from her, but instead are asking her to engage differently.

In this case, guided imagery and discussing her situation, was enough of a shaman's journey for her to experience that past lives exist and those actions can be healed and new behaviors can be formed. "You are learning to find a new way to make peace, create harmony, and still have your own power. Your roommates are worthy adversaries to help you, and you are helping them come to this new way of being in the world without patriarchal, top down, structures." She was able to hear what I said for the first time in this session. She got it. She could see that she was learning *with* them necessary new behaviors. Then I added, "This is about 'power with', rather than 'power over'," [as Riane Eisler stated in her book, "The Chalice and the Blade". (Harper Collins, 1987)]. At that moment she could see that she was working things out, not being attacked and she walked away with a new set of tools, understandings and sense of what might be possible in her world with roommates and her job.

You could say Energy Medicine is modern day shamanism with different tools for transformation. However, no matter what method you are using, transformation happens! And that is the point of working with energy in the first place, to help people transform to healthier lives whether you consider yourself an energy medicine practitioner, a healer, therapist or a shaman.

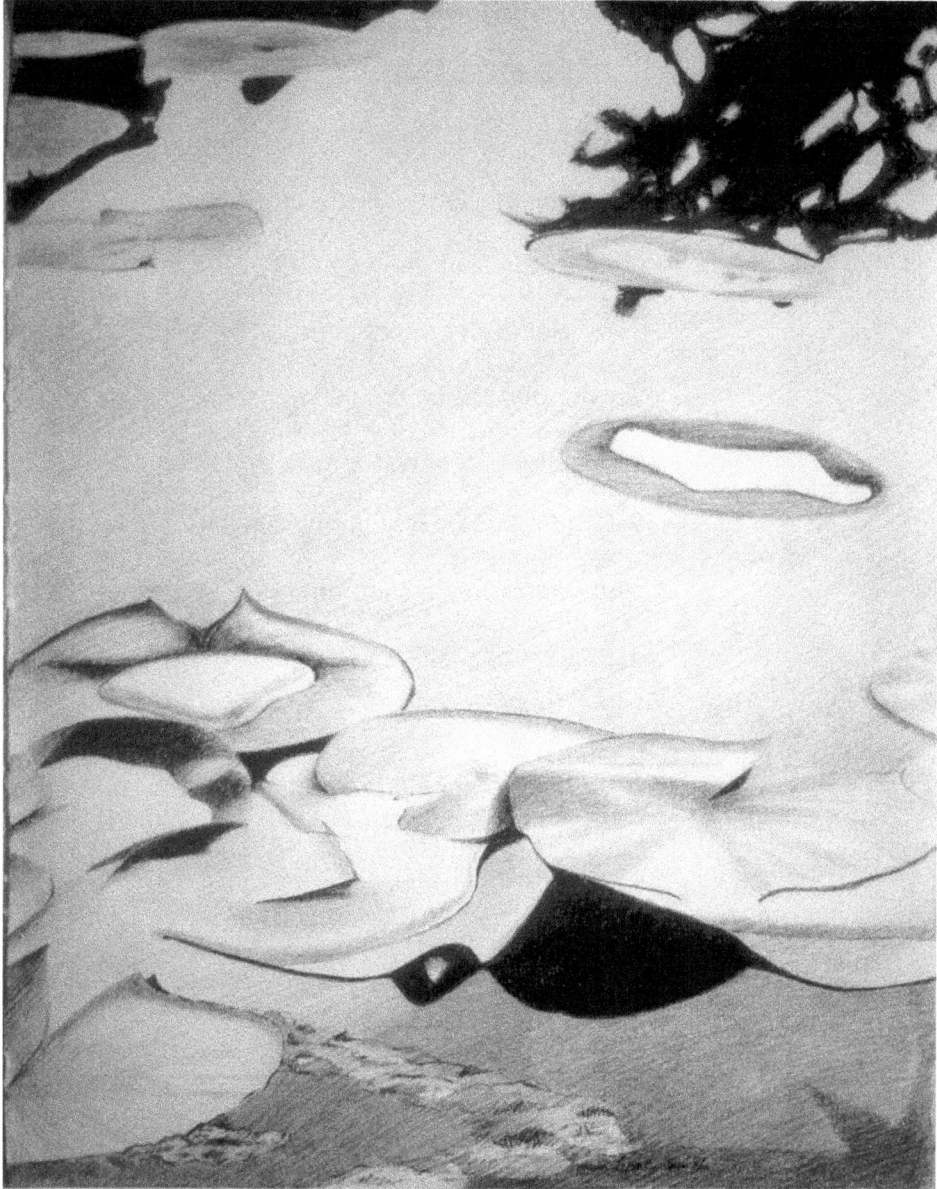

Underwater Lilies - Charcoal Paintings
by the Author

Chapter 5 -Working with the Energy Field

Jasmine Pearl

Enter the tea house where

burls of maple slabs have been

made into tables, the tops carved and polished.

Hot water pours

over the Buddha by the server,

over the cup to warm it,

as swirls spiral down a hidden drain

and match maple shimmer.

The steaming cup in my hand

is full of fragrance.

As I sip the tea, inhale the scent,

I see in my cup

a woman from a small Chinese village

whose job it is to

lay out flower petals over leaves

to infuse them over and over.

She then rolls these very green tea leaves

carefully into pearls,

hundreds of pearls an hour.

Snapshots of her unwind with the fragrance.

Her labor is inhaled

with the Jasmine scent.

I taste her anger and her love. Feel her longing.

I taste mine too.

We are awash in a hot sea of flowers.

A sea between, a sea of longing

We are awash in a sea of hot love.

If you have any sense perception at all—and everyone does—there are several ways you can use this perception to help others. First of all, let me begin this section by saying that sense perception builds on those senses that we already have namely, sight, smell, touch, feelings, hearing, and knowing. They are known in psychic work as clairvoyant, clairsentient, and clairaudient, for seeing, feeling and hearing respectively. The words come from the French, and means "clear sighted, feeling, or hearing."[30]

However, many people get stuck on wanting clear vision with regards to these perceived 'super-natural' sense perceptions. I disagree here, as I experience people all the time that have one sense or the other operating on overdrive and they have been usually born that way. Often they have come into other of these abilities as they have developed spiritually. What I know after being a professional psychic/medium as well as an energy medicine practitioner scanning energy fields and perceiving other's energy for many years is that ALL people have some sort of sense perception beyond their physical senses. They have an animal nature, which is instinctive in any case. Sometimes they often have the most profound sense perception there is—that is 'just knowing.' Gut feelings are profound. Often people discount them. This knowing sense or 'gut feeling' brings us tremendous information if we listen to it. However, most people don't listen. When you are listening, miracles do happen. It is clear to me that everyone has some sense perception. Many of my clients 'check-in' with me to test their perceptions. They use me as someone who confirms what they perceive.

Scanning Energy with your sense perception

After we have discussed what the client needs, often scanning energy fields is the way I begin a session to gather information about the client's situation. Granted, people come to me because of my ability to perceive energy fields. However no matter what method of perception, or what form of perception, scanning can be used every time to see where a person might be blocked and how you can help them with it.

---

30   The Oxford American Dictionary, Oxford University Press, England, 2005, p 312

Scanning the Energy Field Exercise:

Scanning begins with permission. Once obtained, then begin at the top of their heads and imagine a flat plane of laser light from your third eye starting above the top of their heads and moving through their body at cross-section. Go all the way down to their feet. Scan the entire field from about three feet from around their bodies. You may perceive blips or dense energy where there is a blockage. You can also get this information by asking them how they are doing today, etc. While I always begin with checking in with them verbally, often you will get another layer of information if you just perceive them the way they are with this technique. Often I close my eyes, while I do this, and it works to perceive even more clearly. Then I take a mental note of the blockages.

Once the client is settled in, you can ask permission to scan them, or you can direct them to scan themselves. The client will feel it when you scan them, so it is very important to ask permission. You will know best how or if you can integrate these techniques into your practice. If you are a psychologist, you may not want to offer this to your clients however you will know what works and what doesn't with the client population you maintain or attract.

Once the scan is over, you can suggest they go into the heart garden to look at the energy blocks or hot spots. Just bringing the energy to the outside of the Heart Garden, usually releases it when I ask the client what they perceive and what is needed to release the energy. Often, I ask what colors the energy is, how big, etc, as we send the energy love. This helps to 'measure it' and make it less scary.

All the time I am working with a client it is essential that I stay calm, neutral, and playful, without being disrespectful. This helps them feel they can move the energy stuck in their fields rather than becoming fearful or holding on to it. Often I scan their field at the beginning of the session and then at the end to share with them the difference between when they arrive and when they leave. Most all of the time, there is a great deal of difference between the beginning of the session and the end. Sometimes there is a part of them that has created the blockage. This aspect might be a child, teenager or part of them from their earlier adulthood. I often ask; "What is their intention in creating this energy?" "Do they see that it doesn't help?" "Are they willing to stop it?" Then usually they are willing to bring that aspect into the Heart Garden to release the pattern into the fire. Sometimes the inner family has to forgive that aspect and grow them up to current time, then as they grow up, stepping into the inner feminine or masculine as the case maybe. This blending process happens spontaneously as the person integrates and brings their energies to coherence.

Sometimes I share all of what I see, and sometimes I don't depending on the client and what I intuit. Most of the time, I report the scan as I perceive it. I might report that; "I see your energy is stagnant, blocked or knotted here, here or here." Usually we end up addressing everything, as we take one thing at a time and handle it. This gives a less threatening perceptual report. Sometime I see hot places as though there are embers in the field. This often (not always) indicates some disease in the person. Since I never diagnose, I often ask them if they perceive this energy wherever it is in their bodies. I work with them emotionally, and help them clear it. However, unless it resonates with them, and corresponds to their experience, often I will note it, and address it later in the session or next time and watch what happens as they process in the heart garden. Often, just bringing them into their center and aligning with the three stars, loosens their blockages and shifts the energy. Then the work of clearing or releasing the energy of the block can begin more easily. Very often all the blocks, shadows or challenges I see in the field are resolved at the end of our time together. If not, I let them know and often set up another appointment with them to clear what might be left.

If the blockage or wound remains, some questions I might pose are; "Does this blockage relate to an emotion?" or "How about a past or current relationship?" I will also ask them if they have seen a doctor lately that can help them with this if it is not clear after the session. Often, what I perceive as disease is early, and often undetectable by current modern methods of allopathic medicine for finding cancer, ulcers, or other diseases. Unless the illness has been going on for some time, the client can turn it around when it is brought to their awareness by addressing emotions they may have over particular issues. When you handle the emotion around the perception often the person releases the potential for the disease. I would also see if there is a belief that is unnecessary when you work with them around the energy.

Release and Integration after the Scan:

Sometimes I work backwards, giving the client full permission not to let go. I might say, "I am not here to convince you to release that belief, it must have protected you for a long time." (Often they relax). "However, did you know that fear only attracts what it is you don't want? So if you are afraid, you are not helping yourself." That is often a revelation. They are usually hanging on to the belief out of fear.

The following drawings illustrate what I have seen in some energy fields. They also show the resolution after working with the people and how the resolution changes the field. Without a doubt, it would also release the possibility of disease that could form from such configurations in the energy field. While I have drawn these figures in the nude, I do not perceive the nakedness in clients when I work with them! I was merely expressing the vulnerability of such a state and the clarity of the changes. In addition, the blue color shown on some of the pictures shows the enlightened state of a person in evolutionary process towards their full realization. The blue being below is corresponding to Krishna, Star Woman or Ka, the Egyptian Goddess of creation.

More ways to Work through Scanning

Another useful technique with scanning is to gather aspects or energies with the same issue and deal with them all at once. This is done by first bringing all the parts of the self to the front of the Heart Garden together with the same issue. Sometimes there can be many such aspects from this life and other lifetimes. For example: A client has fear of the future that started at a young age. They may have formed a belief around this; "The future is unsafe." What the ego does is to create situations to prove that this is true over and over reinjuring the client with their own faulty belief system at various ages at an attempt to prove that this aspect is right. Once gathered, begin with the youngest aspect. Usually they are the one that created the belief in the first place. Ask them gently what they believed about the situation. Then ask them if they see that it is not working for the person now? Then see if you can: a) have them place the belief into the fire, b) grow the child up to the next age and see if there are any additional belief systems adding onto the originating belief by the next older ages of children. Keep going through the ages until present time. Consolidate the energy into one person at a particular age, that is by growing up the younger ones and have them merge into the older child then the next older and so on. Something else that works is to consolidate the energy into a central ball and then send the ball love. Depending on the person, you might follow the lead of the client and see what perceptions or insights they might have about the energy presented. Once again, energy cannot be created or destroyed, but it can be transformed. For the purposes of transformation, Heart Path can move the energy and transform it into neutral energy useful for the client. Once the beliefs are released, and the child aspects are in current time, make sure that forgiveness of the child aspects has taken place, or there may be lingering resentment of the self towards those aspects that created the belief. Self forgiveness, and forgiveness of others in the circumstances that prompted the erroneous beliefs, completes most healing sessions.

WuLan has stated repeatedly throughout the classes that I have taught with him, and throughout the first *Heart Path* book, that beliefs are not necessary. That goes for religious beliefs as well as beliefs we acquire due to injuries we have in childhood or as adults. We have a tendency in this culture to expect that a belief is something we should count on. However, beliefs tie us and constrict us into believing something that is not necessarily true for all time. Love, on the other hand, allows one to be the way one is unconditionally without the straightjacket of limiting beliefs.

Beliefs are not necessary to have morality because love is inherently moral. Love lets others be who they are, and allows for all people to be themselves. It also sets boundaries with others automatically when someone crosses our boundaries. Love can say no and it does, not only to set clarity in relationships, but also to stop abuse.

Making Clearer Connections with Others - Cording

Sometimes relationships based on attachment are confused with relationships of love. Often there is love in those relationships, but it is predominated with attachment. Literally there are cords attached from one person to another that energetically look like ropes. When they come from one person to the other, they often have a hook on the ends that seeks to 'hook into' another person. These hooks usually have a corresponding "eye" in the client, which is how we get hooked in the first place. Our ego "I" is operating and we attract those who make us aware of that place in ourselves through their "hook." When you or your client perceives a relative or friend hooking them, ask; "Where are they feeling the hook in their body?" Usually the hook goes into the body at a place in the first, second or third chakra level, or power (3rd) , money, sex, (2nd) and rooting or family foundations (1st) respectively. The heart (4th), throat (5th) and third eye (6th) centers also can bear hook and eye arrangements as well as the crown or seventh chakra. However, they are less common unless it is a romantic relationship, in which case all levels will be affected because the heart is involved and the heart affects all levels of the self.

Next ask the person if they see what is written on the 'eye'? It will spell out what their part of the attachment is about. They may get this in a feeling, a visual perception or belief. You can also ask; "What are they hooking you with; guilt; shame; need; want; desire or a combination...?" They will tell you. If they really don't know, you can ask if they want you to tell them what you perceive about the matter. Listen to your intuition carefully. Often if there is a belief by the client that the other person is not able or not capable of taking care of themselves then the eye is needed to maintain the power dynamics. In this way the client's 'eye' or 'I' is maintaining power over the other person. (This is another version of Victim/Perpetrator).

Sometimes a person will come into my office with someone who is acting as the spiritual half of a whole person from the heart up, and the other person is acting as their grounding from the belly down, managing the finances or being the 'earth' for their 'sky.' Together they make a whole person.

As one or the other of them grows, they begin to find their 'feet' or their own 'head' depending on which role they are playing in that relationship. This evolution is what our mothers and fathers often had in relationship to one another. The Boomers have changed all that. The young people today are moving into more awareness surrounding work, relationship and children with more equal partnerships that supports each person maintaining their own 'earth' and 'sky.' It is more likely today that two whole people might come together to have a relationship with both male and female aspects intact in each partner. The current generation is also questioning gender, which should make some interesting changes for people in the future.

Often when someone is evolving from one form of relationship to another, going towards individuation from interdependence or co-dependence, it is important to know that you can shift the attachments and configuration without damaging the love.

If love is present, there may be a time of adjustment, and that time of adjustment can be just that--a time-out for the relationship. Sometimes people I have known have gotten divorced and remarried. Sometimes they stay friends, or go deeper in love with each other. What is important is that as we release attachment, we come into greater love not less love. Releasing attachment helps a person to let go of outcomes and move more fully into relationship with the Self. As one person changes in a relationship, the other will have to change, or the relationship will necessarily dissolve.

When the Heart Garden Doesn't Work

Sometimes a person is so wounded, they cannot 'see' or perceive anything in their heart garden, they see only blackness, or only a blank. Sometimes they cannot go in to an inner place because they are on medication, or have no inner self, everything is external. This happens with people in the Western culture quite often. Their feelings were likely cut off from way back in their childhood and they often go into fear or worse terror when asked to find their heart garden. Often the person feels the blankness associated with terror or extreme loss such as abuse or a terrifying childhood incident. This feeling can be so strong that darkness pervades everything as a protection for the person. I have had a few people go into a panic, and I ask them to open their eyes and breathe. Their ego is trying to protect them from the pain. Their bodies may become stiff or ridged, and they may break out into a sweat. Because death is often seen as blackness, this visual of trying to access the heart garden often puts the client into the discomfort of their emptiest feelings. Panic is a normal response in this case. Sometimes I ask them to light a candle inside and sometimes this works to "shed light" in the darkness.

More often, what I do in this case is to get the client out of this internal space as quickly as possible and work outside with their eyes open. This might be a client that has had severe abuse, or other traumas, there might be some other shock, or terror that is in their history or a series of multiple incidents. While this blackness does indicate some pervasive fear of death, the Heart Garden may not be the way to clear this fear as it brings up too much pain for them all at once. Other techniques of therapy or hypnosis may be better for them such as Gestalt, or even kinesthetic methods of body oriented psychotherapy, TRE or Trauma Release Therapy developed by Dr. David Berceli, EMDR or Eye Movement Desensitization and Reprocessing or Neuro-Linguistic Programing to name a few. They may need to externalize before they go internal. All of this depends on how functional a person is. I have had clients that are extremely functional, and yet cannot go into their internal space due to some kind of trauma. They often exhibit running patterns, where they can't sit still or don't want to stop. They can be externally driven with the need to be in the world all the time. While most often these patterns represent flight from something they do not want to face, these patterns are not always indicators of pathology nor of deep harm that took place in childhood. They can be the way a person is in their nervous system. Sometimes dialog can discern if it is a flight from fear, or flight for the love of freedom. This is to be only determined by the person themselves in conversation. My friend the Ogum is an example of this. Some clients need to move because they are movement themselves.

For more on the elements and their character, refer to the chapter on Orixás in this book pages 11 and 55, or *Heart Path, Learning to Love Yourself and Listening to Your Guides*, pages 65-85.

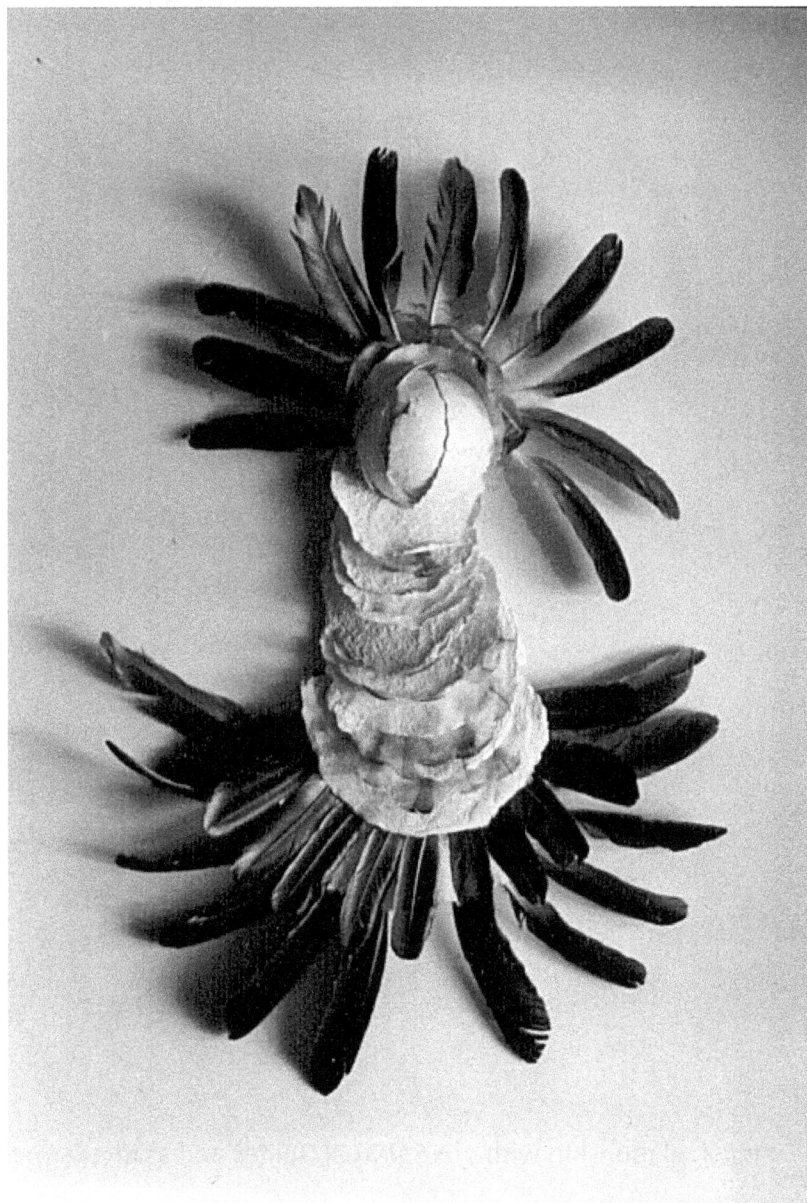

Spirit Dancer - sculpture with handmade paper
and Canadian Goose Feathers by the Author

Chapter 6 - Working with Divine Guidance

<u>Windows</u>

There is a hole to the sky

through redwood ladders

their radiant branches echo

Andromeda's spirals arms.

I watch as my mentor

opens her arms to trees and forests

to all those invisible beings residing there.

As her witness and friend

I stand in a similar embrace

in a oval of bay and redwood

held by the thin whisper of silence

and a crack and

cackle of Crow.

Establishing a relationship with our Spiritual Guides and asking for help when perceiving how I can be of service to the client is an essential part of my work. Because I don't have all the answers, and no one does, we can educate ourselves, we can be helpful, but we don't know everything. That is why we have guidance. They can, and do support the world with collective knowledge. Of course the more you know the more you are able to access greater awareness for yourself with relationships. Your guides also transform energies and might continue to work with a client long after a session with me. Sometimes, I tell the client that they will have someone, a presence, and I describe that presence to them, to help them. Most of the time, the clients are extremely relieved. If for any reason they are frightened or worried, then they always have the choice to send them away.

Connecting to the Guides of Place is another tool available for healers, though few utilize them. This is connecting with the Earth's energies, mountains, rivers, and lakes, as well as the ocean and trees, lightning, and all of the other elements of the natural world. There are whole pantheons of guides associated with these elements called Orixás in Africa and Brazil, as mentioned previously and whole legions of combinations that make us who we are. But that will have to be another book. For now there is a great deal written in *Heart Path*. In short, the Guides of a place live through us, as our bodies are the Earth. Each person can and does relate to the various elements of nature. Some people are watery, some airy, some earthy, some fiery. Acknowledging this in them, and pointing to their balance or imbalance with the elements within them, also helps them to; a) feel acknowledged and seen; b) helps them understand how they can regulate their own energies when I am not there for them. Often I send them to nature to experience and reset their systems to more harmony.

For now I would like to share with you some information that can be helpful about the guides so that you can connect with yours to help you with clients. The following section comes originally from *Heart Path, Learning to Love Yourself and Listening to Your Guides,* and is revised considerably from the original publication. However, to get to know your guides, the meditation has not changed since they gave this to me many years ago, so it is worth repeating.

The Archetypes and the Guides

Once we have a sense of who we are, it is much easier to connect with the guides. However, it is not an absolute prerequisite. Your guides can help you, whether or not you find out about your inner family. Yet, if we do not know ourselves, bringing guides into our being or around us will sometimes only confuse the issue of lack of self-knowledge. We can also ask the guides for help in discovering who we are and they will help us do so.

One important note for those interested in channeling, in healing work, or in helping others psychologically in any way is that it is essential to know yourself first before you begin to try to help others or bring guides into your being. Simply put, if you know your own issues and have healed most of the wounds from the past, you are less likely to project those issues onto your clients or your family. Of course every client is here to teach us something in any case.

Once we have The Path of the Heart meditation down, you can ask your guides to be with you around your heart. Ask for them to come *for your highest and wisest good.* This affirmation is very important, as it is an automatic filter for you to get the best information available. Ask them to come to the edge of the heart garden – outside it. If you feel comfortable you can invite them into the garden. Listen to each one as they greet you. Let them tell you their name, their purpose, and what it is that they are here to teach you. You might want to meet one per day. Some people have a host of them; others have one, two or three. Know that you have the right number for your needs.

The best way is to get connected to your heart first, connect with your spirit guides, and then allow your experience to increase little by little. It is also important to clearly disconnect the exchange or draw closure to your visits. This allows them to be where they are on their side and you to where you are on your side of the 'veil.' The heart is the meeting place of all worlds. This is why people can perceive things through the heart when they cannot perceive things in normal waking life. When the heart is engaged, worlds can become as doors and one can go from one to the other quite easily.

> *   What I would like you to do now is to think about your guides and their qualities. "What do they bring to you?" "What are they teaching you?" "What are they representing; earth or air, fire or water?" You see they can be spirit guides of a particular element. What are they doing? Take a moment to tune in. Introduce yourself to them and ask their names. They may not have exotic names. They may be common names like Bob or Sharon.

They could be aspects of Earth, Air, Fire, Water, or they can be of the quality of harmony, love, announcing, or cutting away illusion. They could be of the quality of strength, perseverance. Spirit guides come to bring you information about your current lessons and what you cannot know about yet in this lifetime. Here is an example from WuLan:

> * Robin has another guide, Xângo. He is the African god of lightning. African *god* is too strong a word…African *Orixá* we would translate in America as *god*. But it is actually a spirit of lightning. It is also

manifested stone. Stone is manifested fire, so the lightning and stone go together. Lightning is fire going through the earth with an electro-magnetic charge. It is also stone, so in the African tradition, Xângo is a very strong spirit that has to do with balance and justice, manifestation and sudden change. He is the god of justice.

"When lightning strikes something it is considered justice in tribal ways, also sudden change. Say there is a disagreement, and lightning would strike and wipe out a village of its houses and the people would have to start over and have to learn to work together. There is a little too much superstition involved in it in Africa. But in any case there is great respect for the element of fire and what that element of Xângo brings.

"Someone else that is very Christian or Jewish would need and require a spirit coming from that tradition. And it may not call the spirit Xângo; they may call it Judith or Moses. Moses was a strong one, he came off the mountain with lightning bolts crashing around him. In another tradition the spirit may be the spirit of the mountain itself--Kali, the mother goddess, who is beautiful on one hand and devouring her children on the other, in the Hindu tradition. All very different qualities, yet each tradition has its saints. They are somewhat similar.

"So it depends on your particular orientation and your pantheons that you feel close to in your life. That is how your spirit guides come to you. And you may have a native guide. You may know nothing in this lifetime about a Native American Indian. Yet you may have lived another life and have another experience as that native person and therefore you have a guide that comes to you to support your spirit." *

Connecting with Your Spirit Guides

Draw a circle of gold light around you for your highest and wisest good. Breathe. Start with your Three Stars and enter into your Heart Garden. Call in your inner family, Mother, Father, Child, Animal Nature, and Higher Self. Create a circle around you in the garden by introducing a campfire in the center or by having a circle perimeter outside that gives you the boundary around your heart such as a fence or a hedgerow, or tree line. Or do both if you desire. Then ask your guides to come and stand either outside that perimeter of fence or hedge for your highest and wisest good. Now ask just one to come to the heart garden gate so that you can get to know it. Look at the quality of light that it brings you. Feel its presence. Is it male or female? What is it here to bring you? Does it have a gift? When you receive an answer or feel complete with that guide, thank the guides for being there. Now ask another guide to come to the garden gate, and one at a time, observe each of them. Ask them the same questions. Observe their qualities. What are they here to teach you? What is it they are learning from you? Take time to be with them across the fence. This is significant for your highest good so that you can be with yourself first and then with your guides. As WuLan has said they are here to guide us not to become us. We must initiate questions for our highest and wisest good, not the other way around. When you are finished relating to them, thank them for coming and take a few deep breaths to return to your heart garden family or ordinary time/space.

What if You don't Experience Your Guides?

Some people may not experience guides. In this case look at what may be blocking the person. You have them, but may not sense them. Everyone has guides. Some may choose not to use them, or even block experiencing them out of fear, mistrust of the spirits or tenacity of needing to know for oneself. None of these are wrong, however, it is good to know which might be the case so that we are able to choose our decisions rather than to live unaware of our choices.

A block to experiencing your guides may be as simple as a belief such as; 'The guides are not real' or 'the guides are merely an aspect of your own personality.' In this case, go into your heart and allow yourself to hold a counsel with your aspects (Feminine, masculine, child, animal, and higher self), see if there are any beliefs limiting your experience of the guides. Release the beliefs into the fire if it feels right to do so.

As an example of showing how people can block what is available, one client had lost his wife in a car accident. He was, at the time of the accident, 45 years old. He was coming in to see me at age 52. The accident killed her instantly, and there was nothing he could do about it. He was not in the car and no one else was injured. He got very angry at God for taking his wife away from him. He blocked out anything that had to do with trusting in something unseen, God, or anything else.

Out of physical pain he came to see me with a diagnosis of a rotator cuff injury from his doctor. We found that the physical pain in his back, neck and shoulder was directly related to the unexpressed grief, as he was willing to cry and release his grief. That was the first session. In the second session a month later, he asked me to call in his wife's spirit so he could understand why she left. In that session, he realized that it was her time to go, that she had life lessons to learn over in the spirit world, which she could not learn on Earth. He actually needed to learn how to live without her, as he had been quite dependent on her. He also recognized his inner abandoned child who was actually the one clinging to her memory.

At the end of two, hour-long sessions, he forgave God and was able to see that he had grown tremendously from where he had been when she was alive several years before. He healed his belief that he had formed when she died that, "life with her was wonderful and life after her death was not." Other limiting beliefs—that God was punishing him for some unknown reason and that God was mean and angry—were also addressed and released. For this I called in his own Guides to explain it to him. Afterwards, he was willing to see his original wound: the time when his mother left the family in his early childhood when she suffered post-partum depression. She had to abandon her family as she was not well enough to care for them. Eventually she returned and was able to reconcile with the family, once the family received the support it needed from extended family members, friends, and from counseling. But the wound of abandonment had gone deep, and he never fully recovered until years after his wife's death when the original wound was reopened and he was finally able to heal from the childhood abandonment trauma. Most importantly he was able to forgive his wife for leaving, and himself for feeling angry about being left. Once he healed all of this, he was able to open to a new relationship and allow love to enter again. His back pain, rotator cuff injury went away, and he was also able to connect with his divine guidance, feeling the Universe supporting him as never before. He could trust God to guide him for his highest and wisest good. Consequently, he learned he could trust his guides too.

In connecting with your guidance it is sometimes helpful to have one guide be the spokesperson for your other guides. This helps to eliminate confusion. They all work together over there, so it helps to have one or two, at the most, that talk to you or your client.

Everyone has a main guide that is with them for their whole lives. These are the ones, like WuLan for me that will always be there. Other guides you have today may not be the guides you have tomorrow. Some guides come in for certain interactions and messages. This happens when we are in transition. An example of this is when we are coming into something new, a change or new part of our journey. Often, if we have Christian background or orientation, Gabriel will come in. Gabriel is the one who announces changes. He comes in with a horn, a long horn, and blows it to herald the changes. In my classes, when Gabriel came through me, he would often blow his horn, then come into a dialog about the coming changes for one person or another. He would come in and announce the coming changes in the world. Every time, he was right on. The next day, or next week, we would be noticing that we were in the process of it, just as he had spoken about them.

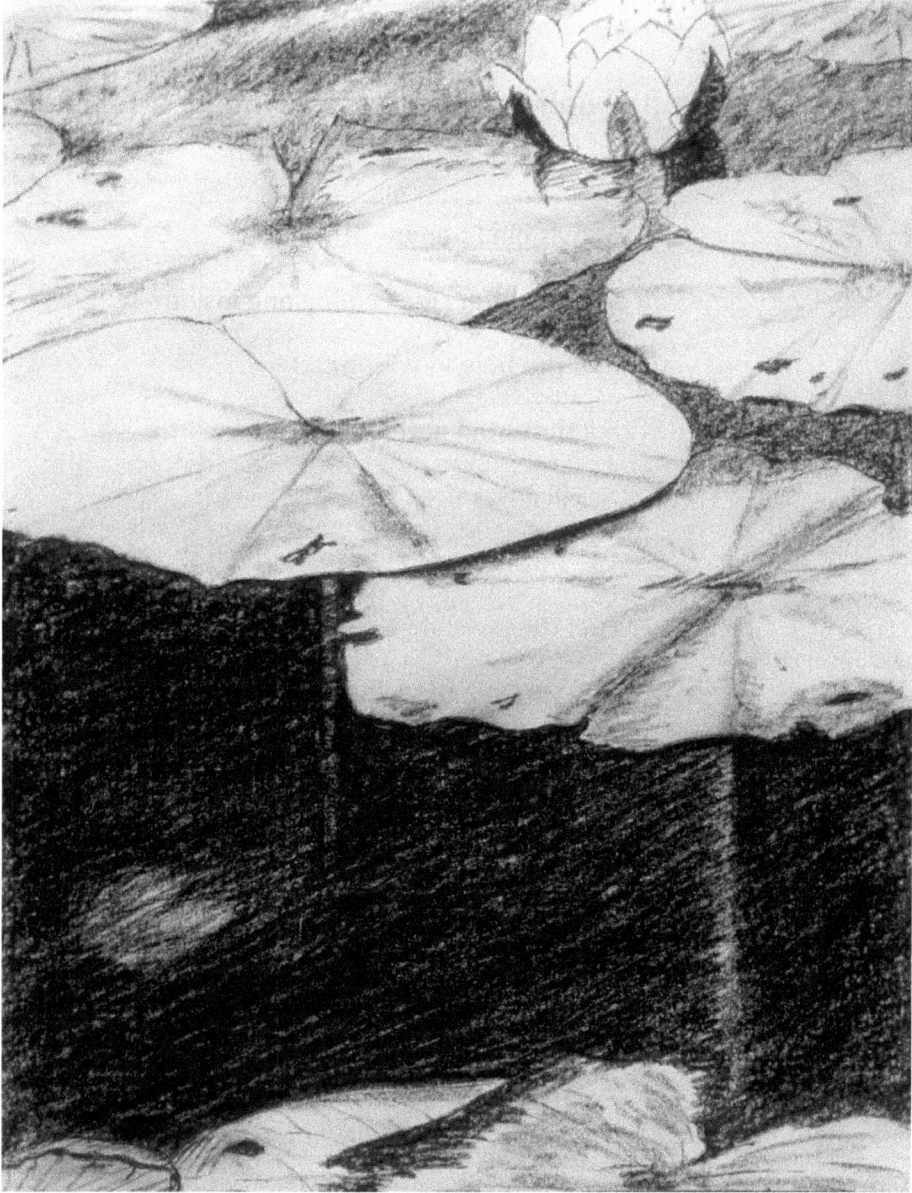

Planes above, Planes below - Charcoal painting
by the Author

Chapter 7

A Word about the Path of Self-Realization and Finding a Teacher

<u>Invisible Friends</u>

Every time you embrace that small crying one inside

you mend the hole in your heart

from a thousand accidents.

Fill and soften

now friend.

Feel the invisible air

hold you in a miracle

as a gentle snow, cool and lacy,

this drifts around you all the time,

reminding you each moment,

how abundantly you are embraced.

At a certain point in development of anyone working with Heart Path, the Inner Family dissolves into the Higher Self, or the Higher Self is perceived as being a Buddha, a Christ-Self, or any other High God-Centered being with whom one is connected. This happens spontaneously as a result of devotion, which is demonstrated by a client bringing the shattered aspects home to the Heart Garden — a literal return to the Heart — or working on the self and transforming into Self. Sometimes a teacher appears before this transition, which is a good thing. I have had teachers all my life, some of whom I would still count as teachers today. It is wise to have someone guiding you through this process and there are always beings that are higher and wiser than we. Some of my teachers have been and still are; Amma, the late Da Free John, WuLan, Star Woman, and others from the past are Jeantte

Snyder, Michael Silverman, Brenda Morgan, Tina de Sousa (Mai Tina), Carlos (Pai Bubi) de Sousa, the late Buck Ghost Horse, Jeremy Taylor, Brian Swimme, Ph.D., Star Hawk, Louisa Tiesch and many others. I am grateful to all of them. Currently and for the rest of my life, I have Paramahansa Yogananda and the entire grop of his teachers including: Jesus Christ, Babaji Krishna, Lahari Moheshi, and Sawmi Sri Yukteshwar. Also Swami Kriyananda, who brought Yogananda's teachings to much of the world.

This transition of self into Self has happened to me, and it is a process that keeps occurring as I go deeper into the Self. It has also happened to several clients that I have been working with over time. Often what precedes the 'break-through' is a crisis, one where you feel as though you are dying. This is ego death. Once the transition is made, the person will feel a sense of vastness. My poem called "The Golden Bell" expresses this moment of self into Self when it occurred for me the first time.

The Golden Bell

So this is what it's like
One moment fear
the next vastness.

Goals cease to be goals
Instead a star-filled night
fills me.

Star Woman
you are me now
as you are every one.

No fear

now love

no contraction   now immensity

I am a dark night full of stars

Yet this is no night,

only shining,

no stars without immense space.

This spot called Earth

one elegant teacher of each

jasmine flower

every scratch of

bird to its

flea bitten wing.

Stop, look how pink is sprayed through the rattan shade

as the copper sun lowers in the west

open to a single hum

a golden bell

calling one

to velvet

silence.

The transition for me was somewhat terrifying in the moment, though the aftermath was defniately worth it. When I was in that crisis point, spontaneously I was called by two of my teachers on the same day prior to the breakthrough. I don't know how either of them got my phone number. But it was their reassurance that I was okay, that helped me through it. Soon after their calls, I broke into a sense of space like I had never known before. I was liberated! Since that time, I have gone in and out of that experience and now it has stabilized into a state of unconditional love, permeating me through and through all time and space. Still there are aspects of ego that arise. I am still learning, and still very human. Though the "I" is no longer, it is self as Self, when fear arises, the response is the same as anyone else. I contract! But those contractions are less and less, and shorter and shorter.

While this is important transition, no doubt, what I have also discovered is that the work is not over. Still fragments of ego that feel separate from the rest of us, left out, not included, can be revealed and released or transformed as we move through our daily lives. Working on the self to heal into the bigger love Self as Love, continues to be a process perhaps as long as we have bodies. For many of my clients, and for me, keeping a humble attitude is key. We do not arrive anywhere, we are here already! Just enjoy each moment. Each moment is all we truly have in any case, no past and no future, no thing or aspect is separate from the reality of the One. As Rumi so aptly put it; when we dive deeply into this moment, "We come up into the fire of being and it is our water...." Each time we dissolve the self into Self, we come into more of our true nature. That is our unconditionally loving self.

I have also discovered that I become more objective about clearing issues. They have little content, and more often it is like taking off layers of armor or dissolving the slings and arrows of my past.

Having teachers helps guide the process and at certain stages it is essential to our well being and understanding of what is going on inside. Sometimes we grow beyond our teachers and then we must leave and be with ourselves hopefully in some sort of community with or without a new teacher. Once we have moved along the path through this state of being described above, companions on the path become as important as our teachers. We move into a state of wisdom and are able to share that state with those that are around us.

Each of us has to decide who our teachers are and who they are not. I know for myself they have changed through the years. Some have passed on, some still work with me on the other side, and always there are those who are more advanced than we are. Sometimes we form a direct knowing about what we need and are guided by our divine self. As we evolve, this knowing is our water our river, our flow of life and that guides us. As Buddha says; believe nothing, no matter where you read it or who said it, unless it agrees with your own reason and your own common sense."

On that note, I wish WuLan, my Tibetan guide, to have the last word. This came through from him quite recently in a monthly meditation that I hold twice a month.

* "Tonight I want to talk about Grace. What is it, and how humans' feel/perceive grace.

First of all I want to say that the grace is falling all around you all the time. It is like a constant warm snowfall that is available to everyone. You only have to tune into it.

"Grace is a phenomena of being in the earth plane. It is where you are held and helped in the arms of divine love every moment. It is like sunlight, radiant and as manna from heaven. It is what the biblical story of manna is all about, grace, the very substance of the universe that helped the people in a time of change and crisis. It can help you as well, every day!

"There are four conditions for grace to be felt:

1) Receiving

2) Desire to be one with All-That-Is

3) Connecting with nature

4) Awareness that the angels and guides are real. This can be a teacher you once had on

earth such as a guru or loving teacher, a parent or relative that has transitioned that you feel around you from time to time.

5)   Faith

"The first condition is that you trust life enough to open to receive grace. That is to allow your self to receive. To open to this grace, sit in meditation, be present with yourself and then feel the lightness falling all around you. It could come from upwards to the right or the left. But just be aware and present. Settle. When you are in a state of rest, when you can let go of your busy mind for just a moment, this is when you can feel it. As you support the conditions for grace to be perceived, just allow. It may take some practice, but this is how you can know the sweetness of grace to be real.

"The second condition of grace is that you have a desire to be one with All-That-Is. This is not a curious desire, but a passionate desire to be united with God, or All-That-Is. One cannot enter this graceful state of awareness without being clear that you have to want to know yourself and others as God.

"The third condition is to feel a connection with nature. Take time out to sit by a tree. Become a tree hugger! Listen and be with the elements of nature. Take tobacco or cornmeal and offer it to a tree. This could be in your own backyard, or in your neighborhood. Stop and listen to the Earth. The Earth needs humans to receive her grace and bounty. If you connect with plants and trees, with a rock or a flower, you will feel grace from it speaking with you. Nature is the most direct way of being with and accessing grace. Sit by a stream for five minutes, and you will feel the love of All-That-Is.

"The last condition is that you must know that the Guides and Angels are real. Anyone who has had a loved one pass, must know that they do visit you after death. You know this through your dreams, through your awareness, and through the graceful moments that occur where you feel them. You might know a bird that they loved, or an animal, and you might see that bird or creature at a poignant moment in your day.

"Here is an example: Robin had lost a sister who she loved very much. Robin was in pain over another relationship, and on several occasions when she has gone through things that are difficult, she feels her sister as a white heron, wings around her holding her. At no time did she think about her sister prior to this occurring. She just suddenly felt the comfort from her sister's graceful presence.

"Grace requires nothing of you, it is truly here, and it is truly yours if you are sincere. This is the key. You cannot feel the grace without being sincerely desirous of feeling more connection to All-That-Is.

"At last, when one speaks of receiving grace, you must be aware of the fact that you are embedded in love in every way--every day--moment by moment! Your faith in this love must be allowed and felt. Love is all around you, unconditionally loving nature, unconditionally loving air, fire and water. This is your authenticity. You are sustained and loved. That is a fact. Without grace you would not be here. It is grace that brought you here and grace that will bring you home to yourself, to your authentic loving presence.

In peace and love and harmony - WuLan the Tibetan!"

Hopefully being with this *Heart Path Handbook*, may help you guide your clients as well as your own transformations. May you take in what you can, and use what works as it resonates in your own heart. May all beings come into full awareness for the good of all. May all beings become the love that they are. May all our eyes open to the power of love to heal all things.

Bibliography

☐ Aurobindo, Sri. *The Life Divine,* Sri Aurobindo Ashram Trust, Dehli, India, 1977, book II

☐ Berne Eric, *Transactional Analysis in Psychotherapy,* Grove Press, Inc., New York, 1961. Page 4.

☐ Bradshaw, Ph.D., John *Homecoming: Reclaiming and Championing Your Inner Child, Bantam Books, a division of Random House, New York, NY,* ISBN: 978-0-553-35389-1

☐ Brennan, Barbara, *Hands Of Light,* A Guide to Healing Through the Human Energy Field: Barbara Brennan, Jos. A. Smith: Book, NY (9780553345391)

☐ Capacchione, Lucia, *Recovery of Your Inner Child: The Highly Acclaimed Method for Liberating Your Inner Self ,* Fireside, Simon and Schuster, NY, 1991

☐ Childre, Doc. *The HeartMath Solution,* Heart Math Publishers, Boulder Creek CA.

☐ Davis, Martha; Robbins-Eshelman, Elizabeth; *The Relaxation Stress Reduction Workbook.* New Harbinger Publications (1980)

☐ Duran, Ph.D., Eduardo, *Buddha in Redface,* Writers Club Press, NY, 2000

☐ Earley, J. (2009) *Self-Therapy: A Step-by-Step Guide to Creating Wholeness and Healing Your Inner Child Using IFS,* Mill City Press, Minneapolis, MN, 2009

☐ Fillmore, Charles and Myrtle *The Twelve Powers of Man*, Unity Publishers, continuously published without copyright since publication date.

☐ Freud, Sigmund *New Introductory Lectures on Psychoanalysis*[1933] (Penguin Freud Library 2) p. 105-6

☐ Grey, Alex. *Sacred Mirrors,* Inner Traditions International, NY, 1990

☐ Gerber, Richard , *Vibrational Medicine,* Bear & Co, Rochester, VT.

☐ Hawkins, Stephen, Leonard Mlodinow, *The Grand Design,* Bantam Books, New York, pg. 93

☐ Hay, Louise, *You Can Heal Your Body,* Hay House, Inc., Santa Monica, CA, 1982-88

☐ Jung, Carl G. *The Archetypes and the Collective Unconscious.* Bollingen Foundation, Princeton University Press, 1969.

☐ _____. *The Symbolic Life, Miscellaneous Writings*, Volume 18 of the Collected Works, New Jersey, Princeton University Press,1950.

☐ King, Ph.D., Serge, *Huna, Ancient Hawaiian Secrets of Modern Living,* Atria Books, NY, 2008.

☐ King, Ph.D., Serge. *Kahuna Healing,* Wheaton, Ill., Theosophical Publishing House., 1983.

☐ Lawlis, Frank, *Retrain the Brain.* Penguin, 2009

☐ Lerner, Michael, Ph.D., *Choices in Healing, Integrating the Best of Conventional and Complementary Approaches,* MIT Press, Boston, MA. 1993.

☐ Levine, Peter, A. *In an Unspoken Voice, How the Body Releases Trauma and Restores Goodness,* North Atlantic Books, Berkeley, CA 2010.

☐ _____. *Waking the Tiger*, North Atlantic Books, Berkeley, CA 1997

☐ Lysne, Robin, *Heart Path, Learning to Love Yourself and Listening to Your Guides*, Blue Bone Books, Santa Cruz, CA.2007

☐ Miller, Alice. *Drama of the Gifted Child, The Search for the True Self*, New York, Basic Books, Inc., 1981.

☐ Miriam Webster Dictionary, on-line www.miriamwebster.com

☐ Missildine, W.H. , *Your Inner Child of the Past*, Simon and Schuster, 1991.

- Myss, Ph.D., Carolyn *Anatomy of the Spirit*, Harmony Books, 1996.
- Nesfield-Cookson, Bernard, Rudolf Steiner's Vision of Love, Spiritual Science and the Logic of the Heart, Rudolf Steiner Press, 1994.First published by the Aquarian Press, 1983.
- Oxford American Dictionary, Oxford University Press, England, 2005
- Paul, Ph.D., Margaret *Healing Your Aloneness*, Harper San Francisco, 1990.
- Paul, Ph.D., Margaret *Inner Bonding: Becoming a Loving Parent to Your Inner Child*, Harper San Francisco, 1992
- Pert, Ph.D., Candice, *Molecules of Emotion,* Touchstone, Simon and Schuster, 1997
- Psychology Today Magazine, Cover Article; *Narcissism*. August, 2011
- Rumi, *Like This! Rumi, 43 Odes* Versions, by Coleman Barks,1990 Maypop Press, #171 p. 62
- *Rumi, These Branching Moments*, translated by John Moyne and Coleman Barks, Copper Beach Press, 1988. p.26
- Rumi: *The Essential Rumi*, Translation Coleman Barks, Harper San Francisco, 1995
- Rumi, *Open Secret, Versions of Rumi*, translated by John Moyne and Coleman Barks, Threshold Books, Putney Vermont, 1984, p.69
- Rycroft, Charles (1968). *A Critical Dictionary of Psychoanalysis*. Penguin Regerence Books, 1991
- Jamie Sams, David Carson, Angela C. Werneke, *Animal Cards*, St. Martin Press, NY 1991.
- Schwartz, R. C. (1995) *Internal Family Systems Therapy*, Guilford Press, NY, 1995
- Snowden, Ruth (2006). *Teach Yourself Freud.* McGraw-Hill. pp. 105-107.
- Tanas, Richard, *Cosmos and Psyche, Intimations of a New World View*, A Plume Book, Penguin, NY, 2007
- Taylor, Cathryn, *The Inner Child Workbook: What To Do With Your Past When It Just Won't Go Away*, Jeremy Tarcher, Putman, NY, 1991
- Thick Nat Han, CD *Learning How to Love*, Sounds True.
- *What the Bleep do we know*?, Film. Widescreen Editions, 2004
- Whitfield, M.D, Charles *Healing the Child Within, Discovery for adult Children of Dysfunctional Families,* Health Communications, Deerfield Beach, FL, Inc, 1989, 2006
- Yogananda, Paramhansa. *The Essence of Self-realization, the Wisdom of Paramhansa Yogananda*, Ed. Swami Kriyananda, Crystal clarity Publishers, Nevada City, CA.
- Zapolsky, Robert M., *Why Zebra's Don't Get Ulcers*. Henry Holt and Co. (2004)

About the Author

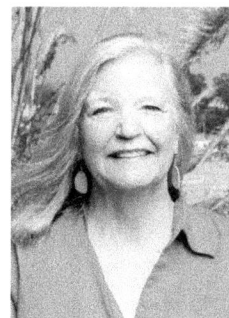

Robin Heerens Lysne is an artist, and author of ten books; five nonfiction, two book of poems, and three novels. Her poems have been published in *Sand Canyon Review, North American Review, Catamaran, Samizdat Literary Journal, Porcupine Literary Arts Magazine, Awaken Consciousness Magazine, Santa Cruz Weekly, The Weekly Avocet,* and other periodicals, and in *Harvest from the Emerald Orchard* and other anthologies. She has been featured reader at Poetry Express in Berkeley, Writing without Walls and the *Samizdat Literary Journal* release reading in San Francisco, and *Poet/Speak* in Santa Cruz, CA. Her poem "First Step" was selected for reading by survivors at the Virginia Tech Memorial Bench Dedication in 2010. Her artwork has been shown widely in the Midwest and on the East and West Coasts. She received her MFA from Mills College in 2012 and her Ph.D. in Energy Medicine from the University of Natural Medicine, Santa Fe, NM in 2013.

She is a owner/publisher of Blue Bone Books (poetry is a cooperative press) and has a private practice as a professional Psychic/Medium and Energy Medicine Practitioner throughout the San Francisco Bay Area and across the country by phone and zoom. She is also known as White Turtle Woman, a name given to her in Native American ceremonies. In addition to participating in ceremonies of two Native American tribes, she has practiced meditation for over fifty years in the Hindu and Buddhist traditions. Her websites are: www.thecenterforthesoul.com, www.robinlysne.com, and www.bluebonebooks.com.

Other Books by Robin H. Lysne

Dancing Up the Moon, A Woman's Guide To Creating Traditions that Bring Sacredness to Daily Life, originally published by Conari Press, Berkeley, CA. 1995, All rights reverted to author, out of print.

Sacred Living, 365 Meditations and Celebrations, Conari Press, Berkeley, CA, 1999, All rights reverted to author, out of print.

Heart Path, Learning to Love Yourself and Listening to Your Guides, Blue Bone Books, Santa Cruz, CA 2007.

Poems for the Lost Deer, Blue Bone Books, Santa Cruz, CA 2014

Heart Path Handbook, An Energy Medicine Guide for Therapists and Healers, 2014, reprinted 2023 Blue Bone Books, Santa Cruz, CA

Mosaic, New and Collected Poems, Blue Bone Books, Santa Cruz, CA 2018

Ceremonies from the Heart, for Children, Adults and the Earth. Blue Bone Books, Santa Cruz, CA 2017

Legendary Ancerstral Women's Series:

The Legend of Randine: Entering the Sisterhood, Blue Bone Books, Santa Cruz, CA 2021

The Legend of Randine: The Laerdal Letters , Blue Bone Books, Santa Cruz, CA 2022

Kisti's Royal Garden, True Stories of the Lysne Family Coming to America - April, 2023

What others say about Robin Lysne's books:

Heart Path, Learning to Love Yourself and Listening to Your Guides, published by Blue Bone Books, Santa Cruz, CA., offers constructive ways for each person to learn a self-love and listen more profoundly to their spiritual guides and angels. Practical methods for spiritual growth are offered, and transmissions from various guides complete the book.

"*Learning self-love is something everyone needs to learn. Heart Path offers readers a way to love themselves without limits.*"

John Gray, Ph.D. author of *Men are from Mars, Women are from Venus.*

Living A Sacred Life, 365 Meditations and Celebrations (Conari Press, Berkeley, CA) "*A celebratory books of days which, with skill and verve, leads the reader to transform daily life into sacred time, sacred space—routine becomes rarified, and life moves from mundane to mystery.*

Jean Houston, Ph.D., author of *Jump Time, A Mythic Life*, The Possible Human, and many other books.

Dancing Up the Moon, A Woman's Guide to Creating Traditions that bring Sacredness to Daily Life (Conari Press, Berkeley, CA)

"*This heart felt book offers simple and effective ways to experience the power of your connections and enrich your daily life. A real gift for anyone who has longed to deepen their connections or experience their connectedness to others or to larger realities...*

Rachel Naomi Remen, M.D., author of Kitchen Table Wisdom, Medical Director of Commonweal Cancer-Help Program.

"*A practical and inspirational guide for using ritual and ceremony to support the mystery and joy of daily life, taking it out of the ordinary and into the extraordinary.*"

Angels Arrien, Ph.D. author of The Four-Fold-Way and Signs of Life.

"*I loved your book...There is never enough of this kind of inspired material!*"

Z. Budapest, author of The Grandmother of Time and Grandmother Moon.

Legendary Ancestor Series: Book One and Two

The Legend of Randine, Entering the Sisterhood, and The Laerdal Letters

Robin Lysne transports us to nineteenth century Norway in this beautifully written story of the spirited midwife Randine. I admired this atmospheric and carefully researched historical novel immensely.

Elizabeth McKenzie

author of The Portable Veblen

Santa Cruz, CA

The Legend of Randine is filled with surprising discoveries. Through the multiple uncertainties of Norway in transition, Randine finds her survival and acceptance tied with a sisterhood of midwives who assist women through the dangers and joys of childbirth using time-honored skills and caring. Randine's life story could be that of many women of early 1800's Norway. Losses, chance and unlikely opportunities coincide with complex people in her life to engage the reader through a rich landscape of a time otherwise hidden to us.

Ralph Knudson, M.D. and Musician

LaCrosse, WI

My own Norwegian ancestry initially drew me to *The Legend of Randine*, and I was quickly engaged by the story of Randine. I highly recommend this beautifully written novel, not only for its compelling characters, but also for its previously untold drama of the development of midwifery in rural Norway.

Ruth Olsen Saxton

Professor Emerita of English

Mills College

Oakland, CA

The Legend of Randine begins the fascinating life of a young woman, called to be a midwife in the first half of the 1800's. It's accurate detail and pace sweeps one along in a stirring story based on historical fact with a gripping narrative.

Nan Heerens-Knudson, M.A., P.A.

Playwright, Actress and Artist

LaCrosse, WI